The Perimenopause Survival Guide

The Perimenopause Survival Guide

MAKE SENSE OF YOUR SYMPTOMS
AND BUILD YOUR PERSONALIZED
TREATMENT PLAN

Heather Hirsch, MD, MS, MSCP

FOREWORD BY AVRUM BLUMING, MD, MACP

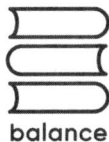

balance

NEW YORK   BOSTON

Balance
Hachette Book Group
1290 Avenue of the Americas
New York, NY 10104
GCP-Balance.com
@GCPBalance

First Hardcover Edition: October 2025

Balance is an imprint of Grand Central Publishing. The Balance name and logo are registered trademarks of Hachette Book Group, Inc.

The publisher is not responsible for websites (or their content) that are not owned by the publisher.

The Hachette Speakers Bureau provides a wide range of authors for speaking events. To find out more, go to hachettespeakersbureau.com or email HachetteSpeakers@hbgusa.com.

Balance books may be purchased in bulk for business, educational, or promotional use. For information, please contact your local bookseller or the Hachette Book Group Special Markets Department at special.markets@hbgusa.com.

Tables and charts throughout designed by Blue Digital Solutions

Library of Congress Cataloging-in-Publication Data has been applied for.

ISBNs: 978-1-5387-7410-6 (Hardcover); 978-1-5387-7412-0 (Ebook)

Printed in the United States of America

LSC-C

Printing 1, 2025

To my daughter, DeMille Margaret Hirsch,
and all future generations of women.
May we all receive the care we need throughout our lives.

Contents

Foreword, *by Avrum Bluming, MD, MACP*   ix

Introduction: Hope for the Biggest Transition of Your Adult Life   xiii

Part I
Understand the Hormonal Hijacking

1: Can It Really Be My Hormones?   3

2: Perimenopause Myths and Misconceptions   24

3: Assess Your Symptoms; Set Your Priorities   50

Part II
Pinpoint Your Perimenopausal Symptom Set

4: Bleeding 'Til You Drop   69

5: Lying Awake and Worrying   93

6: Dragging Yourself Through Life   115

7: Feeling Unrecognizable to Yourself   132

8: Gaining Weight for No (Apparent) Reason   156

9: The Silent Symptoms   186

Part III
Set Yourself Up for Smooth Menopausal Sailing

10: Targeted Treatments for Solo Symptoms   215

11: Navigating the Transition with Confidence   243

Appendix A: Frequently Asked Questions   263

Appendix B: Resources   273

Appendix C: Fill-in-the-Blank Script for Discussing
    Treatment Options with Your Doctor   281

Acknowledgments   283

Notes   285

Index   301

FOREWORD

I first met Dr. Heather Hirsch through an organization called Advancing Health After Hysterectomy, founded in 2014 at Yale University, where a group primarily of gynecologists had been convened to discuss the medical symptoms and concerns of women going through perimenopause and menopause. We all knew that training in this area was grossly deficient in programs around the world. Indeed, the word "menopause" was barely mentioned in most medical schools—and why would it be, given that the male body was (and often still is) the "normal" body that medical students were taught? Our task was to educate physicians in training and in practice through lectures, published papers, and online educational sessions, bringing peer-reviewed research and information to the frontline physicians working with patients going through the maelstrom of menopause.

As a medical oncologist who has spent decades doing research on the benefits of estrogen for my patients, even those who have survived breast cancer, I was delighted and reassured to find myself in a group of like-minded physicians who, like me, had been frustrated by our profession's silence about menopause. All of us had stories to tell of how it felt to be lone voices in the wilderness, urging the rethinking of the establishment paradigm that "estrogen causes breast cancer," trying to raise awareness of perimenopause as its own pre-menopausal phase, and combatting sexist attitudes that women complaining of severe menopausal symptoms were likely "hysterical" or exaggerating. Even in such a collegial atmosphere, Dr. Hirsch's participation brought an added energy and enthusiasm to the program. She had founded and was coordinating The

Menopause Clinic at Brigham and Women's Hospital while serving on the faculty at Harvard Medical School. As I became aware of the extent of her knowledge, her professional experience, and her tutorial skills, as well as her passion to educate health care professionals, I became a fan.

And then I read this book, which confirmed for me the esteem in which she is held by her peers and patients.

This is one of the rare books that seamlessly blend the author's personal experience, keen observation, and careful scholarship with illustrative examples from women's lives. It is both easy to read—for those wanting the basic information—and extensively referenced—for those wanting to learn more or to use in discussions with their physicians. Dr. Hirsch's recommendations are practical and doable, but they are not cookie-cutter advice guides; rather, she allows readers to customize her suggestions according to their own circumstances and needs. Thus, in the chapter called "Assess Your Symptoms; Set Your Priorities" she candidly writes: "The next part of this book is a bit of a choose-your-own adventure."

Dr. Hirsch fulfills the responsibility of both the physician, whose task is to counsel and heal, and the scientist, whose task is to determine the best available evidence to guide diagnosis and treatment. And she does both in the spirit of *partnership* with the patient, rather than dominance. That is why she is equally comfortable offering readers ways to help themselves as well as other solutions that require working with a medical professional. She offers advice without finding fault or inducing guilt. As you read this book, you feel as if Dr. Hirsch is holding your hand and looking directly into your eyes. And her concern, first and foremost, is well-being and autonomy—crucial matters for the many midlife women who feel squeezed between the demands of their partners, children, parents, and employers. As she writes, "Whenever a patient tells me, 'I'd like my sex life to get better,' I always ask, 'For you, or for your partner, or both?' If the answer is 'For my partner,' I suggest moving libido down the priority list, because nothing we do will be significantly effective if you're doing it for someone else. I'd rather see you prioritize sleep or address brain fog, because those will make *you* feel better—and when you do, you may genuinely feel more interested in tending to your sex life."

If you want to have access to the best answers available now for the symptoms and experiences of perimenopause; if you want to know the best alternatives (prescription and non-prescription) that are available to you as you navigate through this often difficult period; and if you want to partner with your physicians to choose the best options available to you, this book will be a cherished guide as you travel along this phase of life's journey.

Avrum Z. Bluming, MD, MACP
emeritus clinical professor of medicine,
University of Southern California
coauthor, with Dr. Carol Tavris, of *Estrogen Matters*

Hope for the Biggest Transition of Your Adult Life

Drew Barrymore sat onstage between Oprah Winfrey and me and was spilling her guts to the crowd of women in the audience. Drew, who was forty-eight at the time, admitted that lately she'd been feeling "dead inside." She'd recently experienced her first hot flash—on TV while interviewing Jennifer Aniston, no less. She knew she was perimenopausal—that period of time during which a woman transitions toward, but is not yet in, menopause—but still, her experience felt really bewildering. "I've heard different answers from different doctors," she said. Things like: *You're not a candidate for hormone therapy if you're still getting your period; Oh, just reduce your stress;* or, *The only thing I can offer you is an antidepressant.* "I'm incredibly confused and I don't know what I'm supposed to do," she confessed.

Drew was sharing so openly because we, along with Maria Shriver and Dr. Sharon Malone, were taping a segment for Oprah's "Life You Want" series on the topic of menopause. The majority of women in the audience were nodding their heads in recognition and some of them even silently wept. My heart broke in that moment, as it does whenever I hear similar stories from my patients, friends, and family, as well as the women who comment on my social media posts.

Drew Barrymore is just one of the millions of women between the ages of thirty-five and fifty (the average age range of women whose ovaries have begun the transition to menopause) whose health, life, and work are derailed by the symptoms caused by the decline of their sex hormones—which, despite their name, have a major impact throughout the body, not just the reproductive organs.

The result is that women grapple with all kinds of symptoms. Jane, for example, was a high-powered real estate lawyer in her early forties who'd recently become very anxious and couldn't seem to sleep through the night. Her job was stressful, yes, but she'd never had trouble with anxiety. At age forty-seven, Lucy was having a hard time remembering things—constantly leaving the house without her purse; she was unable to easily recall words, and she forgot to send important emails. She worried, *Could this be early-onset Alzheimer's?*, fearing the same thing that happened to her father might happen to her. Her primary care physician referred her to a neurologist, who told her she was fine, but still—why couldn't she remember things? At age forty-six, Cherise began having incredibly heavy periods—so much so that she had to wear super-maxi tampons and period underwear and still sometimes bled through her pants. When she called her ob-gyn, he terrified her by suggesting she might have uterine cancer, saying she needed an ultrasound immediately. The test results were normal, and though her heavy bleeding continued, she never got a good answer as to why this was happening.

The reality: Jane, Lucy, and Cherise were all exhibiting symptoms of perimenopause. Yet because so many of these symptoms can seem completely disconnected to reproductive health, few women—or even clinicians for reasons I'll go through in just a moment—make the link between those symptoms and fluctuating hormones.

And here is the harsh reality: Too many women are left to wonder what in the world is going on with them, completely in the dark about the very normal changes their bodies go through in their late thirties, forties, and early fifties, and feeling dismissed and unheard by their health-care providers.

The Long Tentacles of Perimenopause

There's something else too many of us don't know about perimenopause: As we go through the menopausal transition, the very underpinnings of our long-term health can become more vulnerable, too. The decline in reproductive hormones has clear and important ramifications that affect our gastrointestinal (GI) system, musculoskeletal system, pelvic floor, mental health, cardiovascular system, and even our brain.

With heart disease being the leading cause of death in women, women comprising two-thirds of all dementia patients, and more women experiencing osteoporotic bone fractures than cardiovascular events, strokes, and breast cancer combined,[1] it's vital for us to understand that the entire body feels the decline in hormones starting in perimenopause, and how we address these hormonal changes today will determine the trajectory of our health in the decades to come.

Perimenopause also impacts our work lives and pocketbooks as well as the economy at large. In 2023, researchers at the Mayo Clinic surveyed more than four thousand women who reported having moderate hormone-related symptoms. They found that 13 percent had experienced an adverse work outcome because of those symptoms, and 11 percent were missing days of work because of them. Collectively, the researchers calculated, this was costing the United States $1.8 billion in missed work and $26.6 billion in medical costs.[2] And that's just in women with average symptoms. A study by Dutch researchers found that of women whose symptoms were severe enough to get them to seek care at a clinic, 76 percent said their symptoms were impairing their ability to perform at work.[3] And who could blame them? It's tough to be your best when your sleep is impaired, your mood is all over the place, your joints ache, you have brain fog, and you have to run to the bathroom every hour or two to make sure you aren't bleeding through your clothes.

It's Time for Perimenopause to Have Its Moment

In the past few years, menopause has come out of the shadows. Coverage by the mainstream media has exploded and multiple books covering the topic—including my own first book, *Unlock Your Menopause Type*—have led to thousands of women becoming more vocal about their experiences. This is great news!

The not-so-great news?

Perimenopause has not been part of this conversation—and it's an entirely different animal:

- In menopause, a woman's hormone levels are low, but they are steady. In perimenopause, they fluctuate wildly, spiking one week and bottoming out the next, making women confused about their cycles or, worse yet, not realizing that their symptoms are related to their hormones. This means that how I counsel women and treat symptoms of perimenopause is different from how I treat a woman in menopause (and this is the reason I wanted to write a book devoted solely to perimenopause!).
- Menopause has a clear diagnostic criterion—one year without a period. Perimenopause is much trickier to pin down because a blood test captures hormone levels on only one day, when they are changing from week to week and month to month. The result? Women are told, "Your blood levels are normal, so it can't be your hormones," which only gaslights them and reinforces the idea that their experiences aren't valid. It also delays treatment, which then deprives women from feeling and functioning at their best through the transition, which can last as long as ten years. (Ten! Years!)
- Women are starting to acknowledge and talk openly about menopause. But perimenopause is barely part of the conversation—among women themselves or with doctors who are caring for female patients in this age group. As a result, too often women

are blindsided when their hormones start to shift. According to research published in the journal *Menopause*, 59 percent of women didn't think it was possible to experience any hormone-related symptoms until age fifty.[4] Yet I see women in their late thirties in my practice regularly. The same study also found that when women experience symptoms earlier than they expected, they have a higher likelihood of holding a negative view of their overall health than women whose perimenopausal symptoms showed up "on time."

The takeaway? The more women understand what can happen to them in their late thirties and forties, the better they're likely to feel.

Why I Wrote This Book

My goal for this book is not only to demystify your symptoms, but also to explain how to treat them and why doing so is important to your health today and over the long term. Just as importantly—if not even more so—I want you to finally feel seen and get answers from a woman who is not just an experienced and credentialed clinician, but who is also in the middle of her own hormonal transition. Believe me, I *know* what you're going through.

When I started wanting to throw out all my kids' toys because I couldn't stand the mess one second longer and began getting really irritable for about a week out of every month, I didn't think all that much of it—just a bad case of PMS, right? Then I started experiencing the occasional hot flash, but I thought I must have forgotten to turn the heat down before bed, or I was just doing too much that day and was having a hard time settling down. And because I had an IUD and I had only very light bleeding, it took me awhile to put together that my irritability and the hot flashes I was denying were related to perimenopause.

You'd think that as a woman who has spent the past decade treating women going through hormonal transition, I'd have a clue. Well, I didn't. So, when I finally pieced it together, it only drove home the fact that most women don't see perimenopause coming.

As bewildering as perimenopause can be, there *is* hope.

When you get the information you need to help you understand how this major hormonal shift is impacting you, you'll be empowered to make choices that both relieve your symptoms and shore up your health. You'll also be better able to advocate for yourself with your doctors to get one of the many evidence-based treatments that suits your unique symptom set, health history, and priorities. You'll be fully equipped to navigate this yearslong transition so you no longer feel dead inside or wonder if you are losing your mind, but instead can feel like yourself again.

And you'll be helping to fill the gaping hole in our collective knowledge about perimenopause, which will benefit not only you, but also your friends, sisters, doctor, and everyone who will make their way through this transition with you and after you.

And frankly, it's far too unlikely that you'll be able to easily find a doctor who can help guide you through this transition (although I cover how to find one who is knowledgeable in "Appendix B: Resources" at the back of the book).

Why? The vast majority of doctors—even ob-gyns—receive very little training in menopause and perimenopause. A survey of medical residents in the fields of internal medicine, family medicine, and obstetrics and gynecology conducted by the Mayo Clinic found that 20 percent of residents had received no lectures during their training on menopause, and only 6.8 percent felt confident that they had received enough training to help women through the menopausal transition.[5]

Do these stats make you angry? They make me crazy. This lack of education for medical professionals about a perfectly natural yet disruptive transition that happens to half the population is absurd.

I decided to specialize in women's hormonal transitions when I was a fellow at the Cleveland Clinic and realized that the education about women's health basically ended with pregnancy and childbirth. It's not even that perimenopause and menopause were overlooked—they were completely missing from medical school training. They simply weren't considered important enough to be covered in medical textbooks.

A direct result of this massive gap in our doctors' education is that the average appointment wait list for menopausal medicine doctors is out seven months. On top of that, according to the experiences of the thousands of women I've treated in the past decade, many perimenopausal women see five to six different doctors before getting to the hormonal root of their issues. No wonder my posts on social media get blown up with comments and DMs every day with questions and pleas for help. They are seeking help wherever they can get it and they are hungry for information. Gen X and the older millennials are on the front lines of perimenopause, and they are not taking it lying down!

I am on a mission to do everything I can to get the information, validation, and guidance on perimenopause that women so desperately need into their hands. In fact, I have devoted my entire medical career to studying and treating women's midlife hormonal transitions. As a certified and experienced menopausal medicine doctor, I want to bridge the information gap with clear evidence- and experience-based guidance that both women and doctors can utilize.

That's why I wrote *The Perimenopause Survival Guide*—to help you develop a plan to address your symptoms and protect your long-term health that combines medical treatments—prescriptions, labs, and perhaps even procedures where appropriate—with at-home strategies—dietary changes, supplements, stress reduction tools, exercises, and lifestyle adjustments. Perimenopause is not "menopause light," and it deserves its own road map.

How to Use This Book

The Perimenopause Survival Guide has three distinct parts that correlate to three vital steps for caring for yourself along your perimenopause journey.

Part I, "Understand the Hormonal Hijacking," provides the background information that will help you understand what you're experiencing. Starting with a chapter that explains how the hormones that are waning influence much more than your reproductive organs, you'll learn what each hormone does, how they work throughout the body, and why they have such a huge influence on physical and mental health. I also outline the thirty-four—and counting!—symptoms of perimenopause, so you can start to piece together how your particular hormonal shift may be affecting you in ways you didn't even realize, as many symptoms are surprising. For example, many women don't know that perimenopause can connect the dots between their back pain, their low mood, and their newly sprouted chin hairs.

In chapter 2, I explore and bust the many widespread, hard-to-kill myths and misconceptions about perimenopause: *Aren't I too young to be experiencing symptoms? Does a skipped period mean I'm pregnant? Is hormone therapy really safe?* And many more. Then in the final chapter of part I, I walk you through the exact same process I take each of my patients through. When I meet my patients, I want to develop a complete picture of how perimenopause is affecting them, and to prioritize which set of symptoms they want to treat first—and the questions in this chapter will help you do the same thing for yourself.

Part II, "Pinpoint Your Perimenopausal Symptom Set," guides you on how to treat the group of symptoms you have identified as your top priority, outlining all treatments and tactics that have a track record of being effective at reducing symptoms and bolstering overall health. Some of these will require a prescription. After all, I'm an MD. I want to introduce you to and demystify the many FDA-approved medications that can help treat your symptoms—including hormone therapy, although there are more and more nonhormonal treatment options every year that too many women are still unaware of. I'll also cover the many lifestyle strategies that research and my clinical experience have shown to work. You have many options available to you. Learning what they are will help you engage in shared decision-making with your clinician to personalize your treatment plan.

Then, part III, "Set Yourself Up for Smooth Menopause Sailing," helps you set the stage for an easier menopause journey and also for your best health in the second half of your life. First, I'll help you target some of the stranger symptoms of perimenopause that can start now and linger well into menopause, such as ringing ears and itchy skin. Then I'll offer advice and strategies for how you can confidently take the journey from perimenopause through menopause and recalibrate your lifestyle and habits to accommodate your new self as a woman in her post-reproductive years.

Finally, I'll answer the questions I'm asked most frequently, such as "How does perimenopause affect fertility?" and "When should I talk to my doctor about perimenopause?" and provide a detailed list of further resources, such as vetted apps, books, and websites that can help you understand—and manage—your symptoms.

You'll likely notice that many symptom sets have the same or similar treatments, so as you read through you'll notice some familiar advice. While I definitely don't want to sound like a broken record, I do want you to have easy access to everything that might help you manage your symptoms without having to flip back and forth through the book. I've attempted to include cross-references to other locations in the book where you can find more information about whatever you're facing.

The Perimenopause Survival Guide is designed to help you understand what's happening with your body, find and make shared decisions with a knowledgeable clinician about possible treatments, and know what you can do on your own—like taking supplements, implementing dietary strategies, and making lifestyle changes—that have a proven, scientifically tested track record of being helpful, as well as what you should avoid.

Please let these words sink in: You don't have to suffer through your bothersome symptoms and just resign yourself to a life of not feeling all that great. My ultimate aim is for you to be able to walk away from reading this book with a plan that is going to address your symptoms, improve your quality of life, and help you feel educated, confident, and unstoppable in your journey to a healthy second half of life.

PART I

UNDERSTAND THE HORMONAL HIJACKING

CHAPTER 1

Can It Really Be My Hormones?

Jessica was on her first Zoom call with me for an initial perimenopausal medicine consultation. When I asked her how she'd been feeling, she started listing several seemingly unrelated symptoms: Most noticeably, her periods were all over the place—her cycles had started coming more like twenty-one days apart instead of her typical twenty-eight, but now it had been almost seven weeks since her last period. She'd taken three pregnancy tests, but they'd all come back negative, although she felt bloated and her breasts were so sore that she had trouble believing she wasn't pregnant. I asked if she'd noticed anything else, and she said she'd been feeling more anxious than usual, even though nothing in her life had really changed (except for her periods). The anxiety was making it hard for her to fall asleep at night, and the next day she was irritable, snapping at her partner because she was tired. Sometimes it even felt like her heart was beating too fast and she struggled to catch her breath. Plus, her back was stiff in the mornings, but she hadn't done anything to strain it. "I don't see how these could all be related, but they are all what I'm experiencing," she told me. "I don't know what's going on with me—it's like I'm falling apart!"

Jessica then told me how she had already seen her general practitioner, who referred her to a therapist for her anxiety (who told her to take a vacation); a cardiologist for her heart palpitations (who said her heart was fine); and an orthopedist for her joint pain (who told her to go to physical therapy). Finally, her older sister pointed out that all her various symptoms could be hormone-related. Yet when Jessica raised the idea with her general practitioner, he suggested these symptoms couldn't possibly be hormone-related because Jessica was still having her period. That's how she wound up seeing me for a consultation.

The number of times I hear some variation on this story makes my life seem like the movie *Groundhog Day*. Even though every person who was born with ovaries—a full half of the worldwide population—will experience perimenopause, it's like the transitional period is a secret, but one that is hiding in plain sight.

So Much More Than "Reproductive" Hormones

Why is it the case that so many women and their doctors don't think of perimenopause as a possible cause of the many symptoms that can begin to appear when a woman's hormone levels start to fluctuate?

Part of the reason lies in the lack of clinical education and training, but another part is that we think of estrogen and progesterone as merely "reproductive" hormones that primarily play a role in the menstrual cycle and pregnancy. It's minimizing at best, and harmful at worst, to think of these biochemical messengers in this limited way, because they have wide-ranging impacts throughout the entire body. In fact, we have receptors for these hormones from head to toe—and I will take you on a tour through the body to point out the multiple ways estrogen impacts whole-body health in just a moment.

So, if your perimenopause presents as low back pain, brain fog, and anxiety, you might just think you're stressed. Or that it's generic aging. A lot of patients tell me that they assumed they were coming down with the flu, or dealing with long COVID, because they were running warm, sweating at night, and feeling tired. All of these thoughts can cause you to either: (a) ignore your symptoms and wait for them to pass; or (b) schedule an appointment with your primary care doc, who is also unlikely to connect them to your fluctuating hormones (because of the woeful lack of education they've received about perimenopause). Either way, you don't get relief. However, by reading this book you'll gain the knowledge necessary to empower yourself to correct any health impacts before they become long-lasting.

Too many of us still think that our hormones stay steady until our periods have stopped and we are finally in menopause. This is simply not true. In perimenopause, these hormones are all over the place—spiking one week, bottoming out the next (particularly estrogen). All the tissues and organs that have receptors for those hormones prefer a steady supply, whether it's high or low, and they can handle the normal monthly ebbs and flows that occur for most of your reproductive years. But when your levels become more erratic and unpredictable, confusion is sown at the cellular level—and your body's response to that confusion can be equally bewildering. Since so many doctors don't recognize the symptoms of perimenopause, however, you may be feeling as if your own physician is gaslighting you when they tell you your symptoms can't be hormonally based since you are still getting your period. Or that these things just happen as women get older and you just have to live with it. Or that there is nothing medically wrong with you, so perhaps you should "try getting more sleep or go on a vacation."

Perimenopause is also tricky because it's a clinical diagnosis, one that is officially made by a well-trained clinician who can see the pattern within your seemingly random and unrelated symptoms. Just as there is no lab test to confirm depression, there is no lab test to 100 percent confirm that you are, or are not, in perimenopause. In many ways, menopause is less confusing because it's clear whether or not you're in it—no one can deny that you haven't had a period in at least a year.

If you've had a doctor order lab tests to measure your hormone levels and then given you a diagnosis based on those results, that diagnosis is likely to be false (we'll unpack why in chapter 2).

For example, when my patient Katie came to see me, she had low libido and fatigue along with night sweats and had not had a period in six months. Because her last menstrual period was less than twelve months ago, she and I discussed how she was still perimenopausal, and could still get pregnant. (Perimenopause is a big reason for a lot of unplanned and unexpected pregnancies.) The next month, when she went to see her gynecologist for her annual appointment, he ordered labs to measure her levels of follicle-stimulating hormone (FSH—a hormone that tends to rise and stay elevated as a woman moves into menopause). Her FSH on that particular day was in the menopausal range, so the nurse called to let her know she was "officially in menopause." The nurse made a crucial mistake in relying on just the FSH level without asking Katie about her last menstrual period (LMP). Not only was Katie left to wonder what exactly was going on with her body, but she could have also experienced an unplanned pregnancy, thinking her fertile days were behind her. Luckily, she had a menopause-certified doctor to clear up the confusion, but too many women don't (yet).

There's also been a systemic problem that has kept perimenopause, and menopause, for that matter, understudied: Women of reproductive age were barred from being included in clinical trials for the first several decades of pharmaceutical research. The reasoning for this? The volatility of their hormones was a confounding factor, and the risk of experimenting on a woman who might be pregnant was too great to take.

The shocking truth is that women weren't even *allowed* to participate in pharmaceutical research that was funded by the National Institutes of Health (NIH) until 1986, and even after that mandate, many researchers didn't get the message. It wasn't until 1993 that Congress passed a federal law requiring researchers to include women and minorities in their studies. Still, this law only pertains to research that is funded by the NIH—many studies don't use government funding and are still performed primarily on men and assumptions are made that women and people of different races would experience the same or similar results. As a consequence, we have lost out on decades of research into how a wide number of medications affect women differently than men, as well as how they affect women of different races differently than white women. This list of medications includes blood pressure medications, diabetes medications, and hormone therapy, which has been understudied since 2002, when the Women's Health Initiative—a large controlled study that was designed to evaluate hormone therapy's impacts on risk of disease—was ended prematurely for reasons I'll delve into in chapter 2.

The tide *is* turning however. In 2023, the Biden administration launched the White House Initiative on Women's Health Research in order to "galvaniz[e] the Federal government and the private and philanthropic sectors to spur innovation, unleash transformative investment to close research gaps, and improve women's health."[1] In order to fix a problem, you have to first acknowledge that there is a problem. But still, the net result of our missing decades of research is that the medical community is still majorly uninformed about the unique health realities of women. Furthermore, since the WHI was stopped in 2002—an event that resulted in hormone therapy being deemed unsafe (a myth we will completely overturn in chapter 2)—decades of clinicians missed out on learning how to counsel and treat women in perimenopause and menopause with hormone therapy.

There are certain aspects of women's health that have gotten the spotlight treatment. Breast cancer, for instance. Because one in eight women will get breast cancer, we are all prescribed a yearly mammogram to promote early detection. In contrast, every single woman—one in one—will at some point experience perimenopause if they live long enough, yet very few doctors will even raise it as a possibility when female patients in their thirties and forties come in questioning the very real symptoms they are experiencing.[2] As a result, perimenopausal women are likely to be offered an antidepressant or a sleep medication and told to take better care of ourselves, sending the message that our symptoms are somehow our fault.

The reality is, if you were born with ovaries, your hormones will go through a major change that can disrupt your daily life and multiple aspects of your short- and long-term health. And that, my friend, is not your fault.

That means it's up to each of us to educate ourselves on what's happening with our bodies and lead the way in demanding better care to help ourselves feel better.

The Differences Between Perimenopause, Menopause, and Post-menopause

Perimenopause is the phase during which you are transitioning toward, but are not yet in, menopause. It can last between one and ten years, which is another reason you don't want to wait for your symptoms to go away on their own—you'll be waiting too long! Once they learn the many symptoms of perimenopause, many of my patients can look back and see that their symptoms started years ago—they just didn't connect what they were experiencing to their hormones.

While your hormone levels are declining over time, from week to week and month to month they are spiking and then bottoming out. This variability and volatility can make perimenopause the most bothersome stage in this yearslong transformation all women go through. It is also the reason why the treatments for perimenopause and menopause aren't the same—for example, in perimenopause you may only need to increase estrogen the week before you get your period when it is naturally at its lowest point, while in menopause you might need it all the time because there are no more monthly fluctuations.

There are two phases to perimenopause: early, and late. I spell out the differences in these phases in the chart on page 10, but in general, early perimenopause is characterized by more frequent and heavier periods due to the lowering of progesterone, and late perimenopause by cycles that become less frequent and symptoms such as hot flashes and night sweats due to the bottoming out of estrogen.

It's important to note that not all women will experience these changes in their cycles, especially if they've had a hysterectomy or an ablation, or if they use birth control pills or have a progesterone-releasing IUD—in these instances, you may not get a period at all. That makes it even more important to pay attention to your individual symptoms, as they are your best guide for determining which phase of perimenopause you're in, and by identifying them, you can determine the best course of action to get some relief from them.

The menopause transition is when you have gone between nine and twelve months since your last period. The end of your cycles is near, although you can certainly still get a period—and still get pregnant (unlikely, but still possible).

Menopause, officially, is the one-year anniversary of your last period. It also marks the end of your fertility window.

Get yourself a cake and celebrate the end of your monthly bleeding!

By the time you have been without a period for a year, your hormones are low, but they are stable.

Post-menopause, as its name suggests, is everything that comes after menopause, meaning you are post-menopausal the day after you celebrate menopause. Even if it's been thirty years since your menopause birthday and your symptoms are long gone, you are always and forever post-menopausal. With our longer lifespans, women can now expect to spend at least 30 percent of their life in their post-menopause years.

This phase is also divided up into early and late phases. Early post-menopause is the first two years after menopause—symptoms are more likely to be noticeable during this time. Once you've gone two years with no period, you are in late post-menopause, and theoretically—although it's not guaranteed—your hot flashes and night sweats may have eased. (Although some women do experience them for a decade or more.)

Stage	Primary Symptoms	Hormonal Hallmarks	Duration
Early perimenopause	Cycles start changing—typically become shorter Periods may start getting heavier, with more clots Mood changes (feeling down or anxious) Difficulty sleeping through the night, insomnia Irritability and rage Changes in memory and concentration	Progesterone is falling Estrogen is volatile Follicle-stimulating hormone (FSH) levels are less than 35 mIU/mL	Variable
Late perimenopause	Longer cycles (every forty-five days, three months, or even going as long as ten or eleven months with no period, only to get it and have to start the menopause clock all over again) Hot flashes Night sweats Brain fog Vaginal dryness More impaired sleep—waking up in the middle of the night hot or cold	Progesterone is low Estrogen is low FSH levels are rising	Variable
Menopause transition	Going nine to twelve months with no period. Only once you have been a full calendar year with no period, are you technically "in menopause"	Progesterone is low Estrogen is low FSH levels are around 35 mIU/mL or above (and they will remain elevated from here on out)	Three months
Menopause	The day that it has been one year since your last period—unless you don't get periods (for reasons like birth control or an ablation). Then, you might not know what that official day is and your doctor will look to your FSH levels to determine if you are in menopause or not	Progesterone is low Estrogen is low FSH levels are around 35 mIU/mL or above (and they will remain elevated from here on out)	One day
Post-menopause, early	No periods in the last twenty-four months	Progesterone is low Estrogen is low FSH at 35 mIU/mL or higher	Two years
Post-menopause, late	Has been more than two years since your last period	Progesterone is low Estrogen is low FSH at 35 mIU/mL or higher	Until end of life

Meet the Cast of Characters

As you continue to educate yourself on what's going on with your body during the perimenopausal transition, let's take a tour through your hormones. Once you understand how these chemical messengers play multiple important roles throughout the body, you'll see it makes perfect sense why their slow retreat can have such a widespread and whole-body effect.

Estrogen

Estrogen does a lot of work in a lot of places to keep your body functioning optimally. Estrogen is made primarily in the ovaries and its release is regulated by the brain—particularly the hypothalamus and the pituitary glands. But its influence is felt literally from the hair on your head to the bones, nerves, and skin of your feet.

Why are its effects so far-reaching? Well, you have estrogen receptors throughout the body. Perimenopause can disrupt multiple bodily systems because these receptors like their supply of estrogen to be steady—otherwise, things can get glitchy, like trying to stream a movie when your internet connection is unstable.

And although, in general, estrogen diminishes in perimenopause, it is not a smooth, steady descent. Especially in the early phase of perimenopause, your estrogen levels can have big swings, both up and down. That's why one day you can have breast tenderness that makes you wonder if you could be pregnant, and then bloating, constipation, and feeling blue only a few days later, because your estrogen has since plummeted.

This volatility is also why a lot of treatments that may be appropriate for women in menopause may not work or may need to be tweaked for women in perimenopause.

The further you get into your perimenopausal journey, the more likely it will be that your estrogen gets low and stays low. In fact, when a menopausal woman comes in with her male partner, I point to him and say, "He has more estrogen than you do right now." Yes, men do make estrogen (just as women make testosterone), but in much smaller amounts. That is, until your ovaries' production of estrogen dwindles to a trickle. Then you may become the person in your household with the least amount of estrogen.

To top it off, if all your so-called sex hormones were a group of friends, estrogen would be the one who gets everyone together. When it disappears, or starts acting erratically, the other hormones also start to slack.

Progesterone

Progesterone is best known for its role in sustaining a first-trimester pregnancy, and for regulating the building and shedding of the lining of the uterus. In perimenopause, progesterone starts a slow and steady descent. In fact, research suggests that progesterone declines sooner than estrogen does, and then stays lower than estrogen. Which explains why periods can get heavier and more frequent—there's no one regulating the flow.

Like estrogen, progesterone plays a big role in the brain and in mood. It's a calming hormone (after all, you can't have a newly pregnant woman running around taking risks if you want the species to survive). So, when it starts declining, we can lose those calming effects and we may start experiencing irritability, a short fuse, moodiness, or anxiety. If you're having sudden trouble falling asleep because your brain won't stop overthinking, you can thank the decline in progesterone.

Testosterone

While testosterone is typically thought of as a male hormone, women make it, too, and it also starts steadily declining during perimenopause. Testosterone plays a direct role in libido (which might explain why the thought of having sex is either not occurring to you anymore, or maybe even sounding unappealing right about now). It also helps you maintain muscle mass, which typically declines with age. Since the more muscle mass you have, the stronger your bones are, declining testosterone can play a role in osteopenia and ultimately osteoporosis, too. We also know that testosterone can cross the blood-brain barrier, and that there are receptors for testosterone in the female brain. Testosterone has also been found to play a role in cognitive function in men, although research seeking to confirm the same connection in women has so far been inconclusive (this lack of research may not be surprising, but it sure is frustrating). That said, when I prescribe testosterone, it seems to help some of my patients with their memory and short-term recall.[3]

Follicle-Stimulating Hormone (FSH)

FSH is produced in the pituitary gland, the master hormone-regulating gland located within the brain. It tells the ovaries to release eggs and therefore make estrogen.

From puberty to the start of perimenopause, FSH levels stay consistently low, under 20 mIU/mL. As you get further into perimenopause and estrogen starts to decline, FSH starts to increase because it's trying to get the ovaries to produce more. The later you get into perimenopause, the more your FSH tends to rise. Postmenopause, FSH levels are typically greater than 35 mIU/mL, often between 60 and 100. If you're perimenopausal and not getting periods (for reasons we've covered, such as birth control or an ablation), your FSH levels become more important as indicators of where you are in the menopausal timeline since you cannot use bleeding as an indicator. If they come back as over 35 mIU/mL on two or more occasions, it is a likely indication that you are postmenopausal, or nearing it. (Although going twelve months without a period is also an important indication, too—it's just that some women never experience this anniversary as they have stopped menstruating for other reasons.)

Thyroid Hormones

The hormones made by your thyroid gland—known as T3 and T4— regulate metabolism, body temperature, and heart rate. Thyroid hormones don't necessarily decline during perimenopause, but since estrogen and thyroid hormones are, as I like to think of them, frenemies, they can play a role during this transition. That's because all of them bind to a protein called sex hormone–binding globulin (SHBG).

Imagine SHBG as a bus—when estrogen surges as it often does during perimenopause, it can take up all the seats (receptors) on SHBG, so the thyroid hormones have no way to get where they need to go, leaving you feeling tired and fatigued. If your thyroid is already on the low side, this can nudge you into full-on hypothyroidism, which is why many women in midlife are prescribed thyroid medications but then no longer need those medications once their estrogen levels have stabilized—whether because they become postmenopausal or they start taking hormone therapy, or both. Or, if you are supplementing your natural thyroid hormones by taking Synthroid, you may have to adjust your dosage repeatedly during the perimenopause years when your estrogen is going rogue. I see this all the time as a major source of frustration in my patients, but at least now you have a better understanding of why this might be happening to you.

Estrogen from Head to Toe

While your hormones all have their unique roles to play, estrogen is the one whose impacts are felt the most. So, when your estrogen is volatile, it manifests in symptoms throughout the body.

Hair: Estrogen affects the texture of your hair and how fast it grows. You know how pregnant women are said to have a "glow," with radiant skin, strong nails, and a lush head of hair? That's because they're pumped full of estrogen in order to sustain and maintain the pregnancy. When you're in perimenopause and your estrogen is beginning its wild ride toward decline, your hair can change texture, fall out, or grow thin—this is true also for your eyelashes and eyebrows.

Ears: Estrogen can act as a lubricant, and there are estrogen receptors in your inner ears. When it begins its descent, you may experience a spectrum of symptoms, from itchiness to tinnitus (ringing in your ears) or even vertigo (dizziness, which can be due to an inner ear disturbance).

Eyes: Losing estrogen's lubrication properties can result in dry eyes. Changing estrogen levels can also affect the stiffness of your cornea, impacting how light enters the eye and potentially resulting in blurry vision. It's important to keep up your yearly appointments with your eye doctor to ensure that you correct for any vision changes.

Skin: Estrogen plays a role in hydration of the skin, as well as in collagen formation and skin elasticity. Unfortunately, declining estrogen levels are a big reason why we start getting wrinkles, and why we become prone to dry skin as we live longer.

Brain: There are estrogen receptors throughout the brain, including in the prefrontal cortex (which plays a big role in decision-making), the amygdala (the emotional center in the brain), and the hypothalamus (which keeps your body regulated, including your core temperature—hence, hot flashes—as well as appetite, weight, and sleep). Estrogen also plays a supporting role in the production of serotonin, the neurotransmitter that helps us feel happy and has a hand in learning, memory, and sleep. These brain changes caused by our midlife hormonal shift can take a toll on our mental health and sleep—two of the four foundational pillars of health that you will learn about in chapter 9—and therefore, our weight. (I cover the why and the what-to-do about perimenopausal weight gain in depth in chapter 8 and give a little preview in the "Digestive System" section of this chapter.) Knowing all of this, it's not surprising that having an irregular or low supply of estrogen can have a big impact on our mood, our emotions, our concentration, and our cognitive function. Mental health is also a big piece of the perimenopausal symptom puzzle, and it's one we'll unpack more deeply in the chapters to come.

Nervous system: Estrogen likely plays a role in nerve function, although we're not exactly sure of what the mechanism is or how it works. A lot of women in perimenopause can start to experience nerve-related symptoms, such as feeling unwanted tingling sensations in their arms or legs that can feel like minor electric shocks—my patients and I call them "zingers." Other nerve-related symptoms women have told me about are feeling like their feet are on fire, or experiencing the unpleasant onset of restless legs syndrome.

Cardiovascular system: Estrogen plays a major role in the function of our blood vessels and our heart. It spurs the release of nitric oxide, which helps dilate our blood vessels so that we have improved blood flow throughout the body. It also helps ensure that the nodes of our heart beat in sync with each other, which explains why heart palpitations can be a symptom of perimenopause, when our estrogen levels become more volatile. Heart disease is the number one cause of death for women, and in 2020 the American Heart Association declared menopause an independent risk factor for heart disease, meaning the decline in estrogen that starts in perimenopause and ends when you are postmenopausal by itself can increase your risk of heart disease.[4]

Lungs: Although we don't fully understand estrogen's role in lung function, it does appear to protect against sleep-disordered breathing. Asthmatic incidences and other respiratory ailments tend to increase as women hit perimenopause and menopause.[5] There are estrogen receptors throughout the lungs on different types of cells, so if you notice breathing changes now—whether you start snoring, or get out of breath more easily—this could be another link in your particular perimenopause symptom chain.

Bones: Your bones may seem unchangeable, but they are extremely dynamic, continually breaking down and rebuilding themselves. There are two types of bone cells that participate in this dance—osteoblasts, which build bone; and osteoclasts, which break down bone. Up until about age thirty, when women hit their peak bone mass, you are building more bone than you are breaking down. After that peak in bone mass, the balance shifts and you start to break down more bone cells than you regenerate. As you start to lose estrogen, the breaking-down side of the equation picks up steam, as estrogen stops osteoclasts from deconstructing bone and cues osteoblasts to build it back up.

Joints: Joint pain is one of the most commonly reported symptoms of perimenopause and menopause, although many people—and even doctors—don't know there is a connection between the two.[6] The link likely explains why women are significantly more prone to develop osteoarthritis than men and why a significant number of women who take estrogen therapy report that their joint pain decreases. Thankfully, the knowledge that perimenopause can impact joint health is becoming more documented. In 2024 researchers codified the musculoskeletal syndrome of menopause as "musculoskeletal pain, arthralgia [pain in a joint], loss of lean muscle mass, loss of bone density with increased risk of resultant fracture, increased tendon and ligament injury, adhesive capsulitis, and cartilage matrix fragility with the progression of osteoarthritis"—and found that up to 70 percent of women experience it.[7]

What's the connection? There are estrogen receptors throughout your joints, including in ligaments, cartilage, bone, and the synovial fluid that lubricates and cushions your joints. As estrogen decreases, so can the integrity of these various parts, potentially resulting in joint pains and even osteoarthritis.

Estrogen also has wonderful anti-inflammatory properties, so when it declines, inflammation can rise, including in your joints, making them feel painful and achy. And estrogen improves circulation by cueing the release of nitric oxide, which dilates blood vessels and makes it easier for your heart to pump the blood that delivers nutrients and oxygens to your joints, helping them stay strong over time.

If you don't understand the link between low estrogen and joint pain, you may come to rely on nonsteroidal anti-inflammatory drugs (NSAIDs), such as Motrin and Advil, regularly to reduce that pain. That can have widespread consequences, because NSAIDs are fine for occasional pain and fever relief, but daily use can be harmful to your organs over the long term. In fact, one of the most common causes of kidney disease is the overuse of ibuprofen. It's a big price to pay for short-term pain relief that does nothing to address a major root of the problem, which is low estrogen.

Digestive system: We know that women who take estrogen as part of their hormone therapy have a reduced incidence of diabetes, and what we can infer from this fact is that estrogen may play a role in how insulin functions in the body.[8] This also influences our metabolism, such as how quickly we move food through the gut, as well as what nutrients we're absorbing (or not). Estrogen also talks to the liver and pancreas, giving them instructions on how to break down sugars, fat, and carbs, and where and how much excess of each we should store. It's no wonder that weight gain is a common symptom of perimenopause—particularly weight that settles around the waist, which tends to be more harmful to one's health than weight that you carry in your hips, buttocks, and thighs. That's because abdominal fat secretes hormones that then influence your digestive organs negatively. Excess adipose (or fat) tissue also produces immune cells, such as cytokines, that can contribute to inflammation and cardiovascular disease. The fat that accumulates in the belly has been linked to lower levels of good (HDL) cholesterol and higher levels of bad (LDL) cholesterol.[9] Overall, this is not great news because the leading cause of death in women is heart disease, and heart disease is driven by metabolic syndrome (see the box that follows in this chapter titled "Metabolic Syndrome and Perimenopause" for more specifics).

Uterus: As you might expect, estrogen helps regulate our periods, ripen our uterine lining in case we get pregnant, and keep our uterine tissues healthy. As estrogen declines, you may experience increased clotting and cramping because the uterine lining (also known as the endometrium) and the muscles of the uterine wall are not as well-regulated as they once were. Estrogen can also contribute to the formation and growth of uterine fibroids—one nice side effect of perimenopause is that declining estrogen can also lessen the size, or ease the burden, of uterine fibroids in many, but not all, women. (I will go into depth about heavy bleeding in chapter 4, including other possible causes, and how to address it.)

Urinary tract: Estrogen is active in all the structures that help us excrete toxins through urine—the ureters (which connect the kidneys to the bladder); the bladder; the urethra (which carries urine from the bladder to be excreted); and the pelvic floor. Collectively, these structures are known as the genitourinary (GU) tract. As estrogen levels decline, a lot of perimenopausal women begin to experience occasional incontinence—like peeing a little bit when you sneeze or laugh—or even uterine prolapse—which is when your uterus starts dropping down to the point that you can feel it in your vagina. Estrogen also keeps the pH of the GU tract acidic, and with a decline in estrogen, the tissue becomes more alkaline. At this higher and more alkaline pH, the cells of the GU tract don't function as well, paving the way to more frequent urinary tract infections as the tissues become less resilient and more susceptible to bacterial infections.

Vagina, vulva, clitoris, and labia: As you might expect, your sexual organs are ripe with estrogen receptors, which is why you may experience changes in orgasm, vaginal dryness, and/or discomfort or pain during sex, again because these tissues of the lower GU tract function best at a lower, more acidic pH, which no longer occurs with the decline in estrogen. The technical term for common changes to the vagina at midlife is genitourinary syndrome (GSM) of menopause (which used to be called vaginal atrophy).

METABOLIC SYNDROME AND PERIMENOPAUSE

When you're in your thirties and forties it's easy to take your health for granted. Sure, you might eat more sweets than you should, but you likely aren't yet thinking about how that might be impacting your blood sugar levels over time. Or you might be thinking that an increased risk of things like diabetes and cardiovascular disease is something your mom needs to worry about, but you don't because you are still young.

Perimenopause changes all that. Because as estrogen declines, our risk factors for diabetes and heart disease rise. You can monitor how quickly your risk is rising by keeping tabs on five indicators of metabolic health: waist circumference;

triglyceride levels (a type of fat that circulates in the blood); high-density lipoprotein levels (or HDL, aka the "good" kind of cholesterol); blood pressure; and fasting blood sugar levels. If three of the values on these five criteria creep into unhealthy ranges, you officially have what's known as metabolic syndrome, or a cluster of conditions that collectively indicate an increased risk of diabetes, stroke, and heart disease.

Metabolic syndrome is diagnosed when meeting three out of the following five criteria:

1. Waist circumference: 35 inches or above for women
2. High triglycerides: Equal to or greater than 150 milligrams per deciliter (mg/dL), or 1.7 millimoles per liter (mmol/L)
3. Low high-density lipoprotein (the good cholesterol): Less than 50 mg/dL (1.3 mmol/L) in women
4. High blood pressure: Equal to or greater than 140/90 millimeters of mercury (mm Hg)
5. High fasting glucose levels: Equal to or greater than 100 mg/dL (5.6 mmol/L)

It is especially important for perimenopausal women to be on the lookout for and to safeguard against metabolic syndrome because declining estrogen contributes directly to it. Lower estrogen can trigger the accumulation of belly fat and an expanding waistline. Since estrogen plays a role in regulating blood sugar, when there is less of it on hand, your blood sugar tends to stay higher, contributing to your risk of diabetes. Declining estrogen is also associated with a gradual rise in total cholesterol, including higher LDL (the "bad" cholesterol) and triglycerides.

In addition, with less estrogen and progesterone on hand, your sleep can become more fragmented, which then may disrupt hunger signals and cause you to crave carbs and sugar to perk yourself up, as well as raise blood pressure.

The good news is that by reading this book, you are raising your awareness and educating yourself so that you can make informed decisions to counteract those risks. Knowing how your hormones can impact your whole-body health will help you understand that your elevated glucose levels, heavy periods, and insomnia share a common root, and you are not falling apart. As you continue reading, you'll learn the treatment options and lifestyle changes that will help to keep these criteria in a healthy range.

A Symphony of Symptoms

All these symptoms are enough to make you wonder—why, if estrogen is so important throughout the body, did humans with ovaries evolve to stop secreting estrogen halfway through their lives? There has to be some advantage to the perimenopausal transition, or else evolution would have done away with it—or us. In fact, only three species have females who live well beyond their reproductive capabilities: killer whales, Japanese aphids, and humans. One theory that's been around since the 1960s is known as the grandmother hypothesis, which posits that having an older female relative around allowed mothers to have more babies, because the grandmother could grow and prepare food while the mothers breastfed and took care of infants. And in fact, two seminal studies of populations from the 1600s, 1700s, and 1800s found that when families had a grandmother living nearby, the family had more children, and those children had lower mortality rates.[10] That was when life expectancy was considerably lower than it is now. Since today we're living at least 30 percent of our lives postmenopause, we need to develop new strategies to stay vital and healthy for multiple decades.

And because the symptoms show up in so many different parts of your body—and your life—it can be really hard to make the connection to your hormones. And so, it's very common to start wondering if you have a brain tumor or early-onset Alzheimer's, or a heart condition, or an autoimmune disease like chronic fatigue, or if it might be depression. These symptoms can be *doozies*.

And yet.

Those same symptoms are also typically what leads you to take action, seeking out treatments and finding ways to support your health during this transitional time. Symptoms are driving our curiosity and inspiring conversations in real life and on social media, which in turn is building momentum for changes in the medical community.

As much as these symptoms suck, they are our way out of this. Acknowledging them is the first step in no longer having to suffer in silence. As my grandmother always used to say, there's no prize for suffering.

If we didn't get symptoms at all, we might not realize that our changing hormones mean that we need to start taking care of ourselves and putting our health higher up on our list of priorities. We also might not be so motivated to educate ourselves and advocate for ourselves with our health-care providers. Do I wish every doctor would be educated on the symptoms and treatments of perimenopause and proactively bring it up with every one of their female patients? Absolutely. Sadly, they aren't and they don't (yet). In the meantime, our symptoms are inspiring us to stand up for ourselves and advocate for change.

IF YOU DO ONE THING: START TRACKING YOUR CYCLES

In these first two chapters, when we're covering so much of the background information you need to understand what's going on with you during this perimenopausal phase of life, I still want you to be able to take action that is going to help you help yourself feel better. I'll be sharing these tips to enable you to start moving the needle on your quality of life.

The first practical task I recommend is to get a notebook or journal, or dedicate a Google or Word doc, spreadsheet, or a new note in your Notes app that you can use to start recording information that will provide you with some objectivity and clarity on your perimenopausal journal. Since that's such an easy task, I'm also going to ask you to then get out your calendar and write down the start and end dates of your last three to five periods. Then, from here on out, every time your cycle starts and ends, you can write it down in this same spot. This information will help you and any clinician you may see understand what's going on with your cycle and your hormones.

(And if you don't get periods, start jotting down any spotting or discharge you may notice.)

One of the most frustrating things about perimenopause is that it is unpredictable and thus confusing. Keeping track of your periods won't make them more regular, but it will help you detect if there are any cyclical patterns to your symptoms—which I'll ask you to start tracking at the end of chapter 2.

CHAPTER 2

Perimenopause Myths and Misconceptions

Because perimenopause has been understudied by the medical community, and talked about so little by society at large, there have been lots of opportunities for misinformation, myths, and misconceptions to take up space in our collective understanding of what perimenopause is and isn't.

I've heard some variation on the myths I unpack in this chapter from hundreds of women, either on social media, during my speaking engagements, or in medical appointments, so I know there is a big hunger and a huge need for clarification on perimenopause in general and hormone therapy specifically. Let's review (and debunk!) some of the most common perimenopause myths and misunderstandings.

Myth: *If I'm in My Thirties or Forties, I'm Too Young for Perimenopause*

The Centers for Disease Control and Prevention (CDC) reports that the average age at the beginning of perimenopause is forty-seven. But you can't assume that any symptom you experience before forty-seven isn't hormonally related for three reasons: (1) An average number means there are plenty of people who are both younger and older than that age when they enter perimenopause. (2) Because perimenopause isn't typically taught in medical school curricula, it is widely underdiagnosed, which means it's not being reported properly. Again, it's not the doctors' fault—they're not taught about it, so they don't know how to treat it, making it easier for them to say, "You're too young." And (3) there is no blood test for perimenopause. (That one exists is a myth we'll address in this chapter.) As I covered in chapter 1, perimenopause is a "clinical diagnosis," one that needs to be made by a clinician based on your symptoms and your health history. Based on point number two—that not enough clinicians are educated to spot perimenopause—it is likely that no one is making the diagnosis at the onset of symptoms.

I routinely see patients in their late thirties and early forties who come in with classic symptoms of perimenopause. Again, you are never too young to discuss what you think could be perimenopause with your care team.

Myth: *If I Still Get My Period, I Can't Be Perimenopausal*

This is blatantly false. Remember that perimenopause can last between one and ten years—and you hit menopause only when you haven't had a period in one year. So that means there are generally multiple years when you are still bleeding and having symptoms of either low estrogen, progesterone, or testosterone. In fact, one of the earliest signs of perimenopause is that your periods become irregular. Sure, they may not be the same as they were five years ago, *but you're still having them.*

Every cycle, your estrogen drops the closer you get to your period. That's what causes PMS—the moodiness, the bloating, the fatigue. In perimenopause, your estrogen drops even further, which means that perimenopause is basically PMS on steroids. PMS, as you well know, stands for premenstrual syndrome. Which means you are in fact menstruating.

Myth: *There's a Test for Perimenopause*

I wish there were, because I know how comforting it would be to have a definitive diagnosis, but there just isn't one. Remember, perimenopause is a clinical diagnosis, meaning it must be made by a knowledgeable clinician based upon the patient's symptoms and health history.

I can't tell you how often I hear a woman say, "I went to my doctor, they checked my labs, and said they're all normal." But lab tests that check your hormone levels—typically estrogen, FSH, and maybe testosterone—capture only what's happening on that one day, while your hormones are continually in flux throughout the month. No lab test can rule in or rule out perimenopause on its own. So, to be told you're not in perimenopause (or that you're in menopause), based on a lab test on its own, can be misleading as well as invalidating of your own experience. It can also have significant medical consequences. If, like Katie in chapter 1, your doctor tells you that according to your FSH levels you're in menopause, but it's only been nine months since your last period, if you do get your period in the next three months, it would be inappropriately labeled "postmenopausal bleeding," which is atypical and needs to be investigated with tests that can cause a lot of fear and discomfort, instead of perimenopausal bleeding, which is completely normal. See how far down the rabbit hole one can go with the wrong diagnosis?

Diagnosing perimenopause is like old-fashioned navigation (and sometimes it feels more like detective work). Instead of using the night sky, charts, and measurement tools, we use our clinical experience, your description of what you've been experiencing, your health history, and your period history to make the call.

MY TAKE ON THE DUTCH TEST

The Dutch Test (Dried Urine Test for Comprehensive Hormones), uses dried urine to assess thirty-five hormone metabolites in urine. It has become popular with some clinicians and heralded as a way to get better insight into a woman's hormone levels. I understand why this test has risen in popularity— women are hungry for information about what's happening with their bodies. The problem is that it still captures only one day's worth of information, and your hormone levels on one particular day are not that insightful. A more pressing concern is that without a clinician who has been trained in perimeno-pause to make sense of these levels, you may end up feeling more anxious and frustrated than before the test results arrived.

I do use blood tests to measure my patients' levels of estro-gen, testosterone, and FSH. Ideally, I have my patients repeat those tests a handful of times over a few weeks so that we can see the trend over time and not just rely on what was happen-ing on one particular day—however, this is time-consuming, and even though these tests are typically covered by insurance (unlike the Dutch Test), the expense can add up. Still, those lab results are only a partial factor in my recommendations for a treatment plan. I consider them as helpful data points, but I rely more heavily on the clinical scenario when making treat-ment recommendations.

Remember, no one test can tell you definitively that you are, or are not, in perimenopause. Save your money.

Myth: My Mental Health Symptoms Can't Be due to Hormones

As you learned in the last chapter, estrogen and progesterone have pro-found effects on the brain, so it should come as no surprise that the drop in hormones in perimenopause affects mood. Specifically, estrogen works closely with serotonin, the happy neurochemical—where there is estrogen, serotonin tends to follow. When estrogen declines, so might serotonin, which can then be associated with symptoms of depression. Similarly, there are also progesterone receptors in the brain, and pro-gesterone is calming. When it declines, you may experience an increase of anxious feelings. The changing levels of both hormones also impact your sleep, which influences day-to-day functioning and mood.

While antidepressants and antianxiety meds can help—and are probably the first option your primary care doctor will mention—they aren't the only options. I'll talk in depth about treatment approaches to the mental health symptoms of perimenopause in chapters 5 (for anxiety) and 6 (for depression).

Some women also start to notice cognitive changes, including changes in attention span, difficulty with short-term memory, or finding the right word in speech or thought. Because estrogen is so impactful on our brains, it's not surprising to me that these symptoms start in perimenopause and persist through menopause, but luckily these symptoms tend to improve during late postmenopause. It's not fair that our brain function can get a little wonky during this time of life when our plates are typically their fullest, but we will cover how to address these changes in chapter 6.

Myth: *Taking an Antidepressant Will Alleviate My Perimenopausal Symptoms*

Clinicians who have either been taught that hormone therapy is unsafe or haven't been adequately trained in the safety and efficacy of hormone therapy may suggest that you try an antidepressant, particularly if you come into their office with symptoms like feeling irritable, unable to feel joy, anxious, or fatigued, as these are symptoms that can be the result of either hormonal changes or mood disorders.

There are mood symptoms of perimenopause, and there are mood disorders—because they have different root causes, they also have different treatments. Simply put, mood medications may not adequately address the reason why your mood is all over the place in perimenopause.

That being said, there are definitely times when these medications are appropriate. For instance, they may help stabilize you while you find a clinician who can support these changes with the hormone therapy regimen that works for you, or while you experiment with lifestyle changes that help support your mood. While I'm not aware of your medical history or your specific life experiences, simply put, if you are experiencing symptoms of depression or anxiety for the first time in your forties or even late thirties, hormone shifts are likely playing a role.

The best way to differentiate between perimenopausal mood symptoms and mood disorders such as depression and anxiety is to track your symptoms, ideally for two to three months. If you notice any kind of cyclic pattern or intermittence to your mood—as opposed to its being chronic or worsening with time—that's a huge clue that the mood changes are related to your hormones.

Of course, this is complicated by the fact that your cycle may well be irregular, and you may not even be getting a period for the reasons I listed on page 9. But either way, you could still have cyclic mood symptoms.

Additionally, if you are having other symptoms of perimenopause—such as irregular cycles, declining libido, and difficulty sleeping—this also suggests that your mood changes are a symptom of perimenopause as opposed to full-on anxiety or depression.

For my patients who feel in their hearts that there's a cyclic or hormonal component to their mood and overall energy level, I counsel them to try hormone therapy first because it can address not only their mood symptoms but a consortium of other symptoms, too (such as difficulty sleeping and hot flashes). You can always come back around to mood medications if hormone therapy proves ineffective for these specific symptoms. Some small but promising research shows that hormone therapy may improve depressive symptoms.[1]

You'll find other approaches to supporting your mood in chapters 5 and 6 (depending on whether you're leaning more toward worry, heart palpitations, and difficulty relaxing, which I cover in chapter 5; or more toward depressive-type symptoms, such as fatigue, low motivation, and feeling "flat" or "down," which I cover in chapter 6).

Finally, an important note: If you are having suicidal thoughts, please don't delay in calling the national Suicide and Crisis Hotline by dialing 988. In this case, we don't want to wait to find out what the cause of the thoughts are before getting you some support.

Myth: *If I Take Good Care of Myself and I Work Hard to Stay Healthy, Perimenopause Will Be a Breeze*

Maintaining a healthy lifestyle (including eating well, exercising regularly, not smoking, keeping alcohol intake down, and reducing stress) will support you through your transition; these nourishing coping mechanisms help you to be more resilient during this huge physiological change. Yet, as Oprah famously said, "You can't outrun the menopause train," and the same is true for perimenopause.

Just as being "healthy" doesn't protect you from experiencing things like infertility, cancer, or migraines, you cannot out-yoga, out-journal, or out-juice the drop in estrogen, progesterone, and testosterone.

I know a lot of women who eat well and exercise who feel blindsided by perimenopause and maybe even betrayed by their own bodies. Experiencing perimenopausal symptoms—even severe ones—doesn't mean that you're a failure or you've done anything wrong. It just means that you are a living human whose ovaries are going through their inevitable transition.

Myth: *A Bad Perimenopause Means a Bad Menopause*

What I see most often is that when women have a really difficult perimenopause because of the volatility in hormones, once those hormones start to stabilize after menopause (or when a woman hits one year of no periods)—even though they're low—these women tend to do a lot better. Your hormone receptors can adapt, but it's difficult to adapt to levels that are changing every day, as they often are in perimenopause. Once they get low, and stay low, those hormone receptors can acclimate.

For some women, it's the opposite—perimenopause is manageable, but then symptoms start to kick up and quality of life starts to decline after they go one year without a period. We're all built a little differently. Our receptors are different, and the way they respond is different.

No matter how severe your perimenopause symptoms are, if you seek out treatment and establish or continue health-supportive habits, you're setting yourself up for as smooth a menopausal transition as possible.

Myth: *If I'm in Perimenopause, I Can No Longer Get Pregnant*

This is simply untrue (however, it is very unlikely if you are using a form of contraception). Even though your periods may be highly irregular—or you may not even be getting periods because you've had an ablation or a hysterectomy, or because you have an IUD or are on another continuous birth control, for example—you could still ovulate. And since your periods are becoming more unpredictable, so is ovulation. If you've been using the family planning fertility method (tracking your cycles and using birth control only when you're ovulating), that method is no longer trustworthy, no matter how regular your cycles once were.

There's a misperception that birth control is for young women, single women, or women with multiple partners. In my experience, many older monogamous and heterosexual women think they don't need birth control, but if you do not wish to have an unintended pregnancy, this is false. While the odds may not be high, until you've gone a full year without a period, you can absolutely still get pregnant—something that will be top of mind the first few times your period is either delayed or skipped altogether. If you want to be absolutely sure that you don't become pregnant, I still recommend that you use some form of contraception. I'll cover the many forms of contraception in chapter 4.

While we're on the topic, if you are wondering how hormone therapy influences fertility, it is not a form of birth control. While it won't prevent you from getting pregnant, it also won't hurt your chances of conceiving if you do want to have a baby. Hormones tend to support ovarian function, so it might even help (although it's not prescribed for this reason).

Myth: *Not Sleeping Well, Being More Forgetful, and Having Low Energy Means I'm Not Taking Good Enough Care of Myself*

This myth is closely related to the idea that being healthy and fit will help avoid a tough perimenopause, but it is a little different, because this myth blames the victim.

We place a lot of emphasis on self-care, and that's a good thing, but it is also true that there are a lot of companies, websites, and influencers who want you to buy into the idea that you're not doing the right things to take care of yourself so that you will want to buy their products.

To be frank, you don't have a lot of control over the physiological and hormonal changes that are happening now. Yes, your behavior has a lot of influence over your health. But there aren't enough kale salads in the world to make perimenopause a breeze. You aren't being punished for being lazy or eating processed food or staying up too late, although I know how easy it is to entertain those thoughts (trust me; I have them, too).

Of course, learning to adapt your self-care strategies to your new hormonal reality really will help to support you and retain your quality of life. But women are constantly being given the message that they're doing something wrong. You are not. The fact that you are seeking out vetted information tells me that you are doing a great job at tending to your health.

PERIMENOPAUSE REMEDIES I DON'T RECOMMEND

If you scroll through social media now, you'll likely see ad after ad for products that claim to reduce perimenopausal symptoms, such as over-the-counter progesterone creams, wild yam creams, and adrenal support supplements. While these products aren't necessarily harmful, they're not all that helpful, either. If you've tried them and saw either a small benefit or a noticeable benefit that then went away, chalk it up to the placebo effect. The biggest risks are to your pocketbook and your hopes. Keep reading, because I'm going to offer you a whole host of evidence-based treatments and strategies in the chapters to come.

Myth: *If I'm Having Trouble Sleeping, It's Probably due to High Stress Levels and Stress Hormones, Such as Cortisol*

I see a lot of content targeted at women in their thirties and forties that talks about how to lower their cortisol levels. On one level, this makes sense: Cortisol is an important chemical released by the adrenal glands that helps to keep us alive in the face of stress, especially in the event we need to respond to something quickly and need a surge of energy. Cortisol revs the nervous system and puts you into a state of heightened awareness. So, if your cortisol is high, it can be hard to sleep, hard to concentrate, and harder for your body to digest food and regulate your blood sugar, potentially leading to weight gain, especially around the waistline. Do these symptoms sound familiar? They overlap with perimenopausal symptoms quite closely for good reason—because as estrogen declines, it's common for cortisol levels to creep up.

Why? It starts in your brain—the hypothalamus, to be exact, which is the gland that regulates levels of all different kinds of hormones. The hypothalamus is what cues your ovaries to make estrogen, but as your ovaries start producing less, they don't sufficiently answer the hypothalamus's call. Then the hypothalamus will reach out to the adrenal glands and essentially ask, "What have you got that we could use to keep things running around here?" And the adrenals say, "How about some of this cortisol?" Since the stress hormone is chemically similar to estrogen, the hypothalamus says, "Okay, that'll work." It's like sending a teenager to the store for eggs and they come back with liquid egg whites.

Most of the content that addresses the dangers of cortisol doesn't connect the dots between stress hormones and reproductive hormones. Those same posts and articles may also be suggesting that you take adrenal supplements to help bring your cortisol down, which isn't going to address the root cause of why the adrenals are cranking out so much cortisol. I don't think adrenal supplements are going to hurt you—but I also think they may not be worth the money. Without that connection, the message sounds like "You've got to manage your stress better," which is, let's face it, stressful.

If you're over thirty-five and your cortisol is high, it very likely is triggered by the fact that your ovaries aren't producing as much estrogen as they once were. Supporting your declining estrogen with hormone therapy (and, if you're concerned about hormone therapy in general—I'll address this shortly!) can help bring those cortisol levels down, because then the brain won't need to rely on the adrenals to produce it quite so much.

By understanding the importance of the loss of hormones and why we get a spike in cortisol, instead of blaming cortisol and taking all these adrenal supplements, we can shift the blame off ourselves and our stress levels, and we can look to replacing estrogen as an option.

Myth: *The Way Out of Perimenopausal Symptoms Is to Balance My Hormones*

This is as big a myth as work-life balance. Even before you're perimenopausal, there is no such thing as hormonal balance because as your estrogen is rising, your progesterone is dipping, and vice versa. Once things start getting a little wackier as your ovaries start producing estrogen more erratically and progesterone less as you move through perimenopause, balance is an even bigger fallacy. Instead of aiming for balance, a better approach is to smooth out the spikes and dips so that you can feel and function at your best.

HORMONAL FLUCTUATIONS AT A GLANCE

To really understand why perimenopause can feel like such as wild ride, it's helpful to see just how volatile your hormone levels are now—even more so than in puberty!

There are two main parts to your monthly cycle:

The follicular phase is the first fourteen days of your cycle (or so, this will vary as your move through perimenopause and your cycles change), when estrogen is rising and progesterone is falling. It's called "follicular" because this is when your ovarian follicles are maturing in preparation for releasing an egg at ovulation.

The luteal phase, or the second fourteen days of the cycle (again, subject to change in perimenopause), is when progesterone rises and estrogen falls. It's called "luteal" because during this phase the follicle that just released an egg collapses and is transformed into a temporary collection of cells known as the corpus luteum, which then produces progesterone to help create a welcoming environment in the uterus for a potential pregnancy.

The Hormone Levels over the Lifespan chart on page 36 shows what these two phases look like before you are perimenopausal, what they look like once you are in full-swing perimenopause, and what happens to those phases once you're post-menopausal.

Given the different hormonal realities of each phase, they tend to each have their own set of symptoms. In the luteal, low-estrogen phase, symptoms tend to be of the "hot and dry" variety, meaning hot flashes, night sweats, vaginal dryness, dry skin, dry eyes, irritability, hostility, anger, and even rage. In the follicular, low progesterone and spiking estrogen phase, symptoms tend to be breast tenderness, feeling weepy or perhaps more anxious, and difficulty sleeping through the night as progesterone declines further than it typically has.

This is why tracking your symptoms and journaling is so

important—it's the best way to start to connect the dots between what you're experiencing and what your hormones are doing.

Hormone Levels over the Lifespan

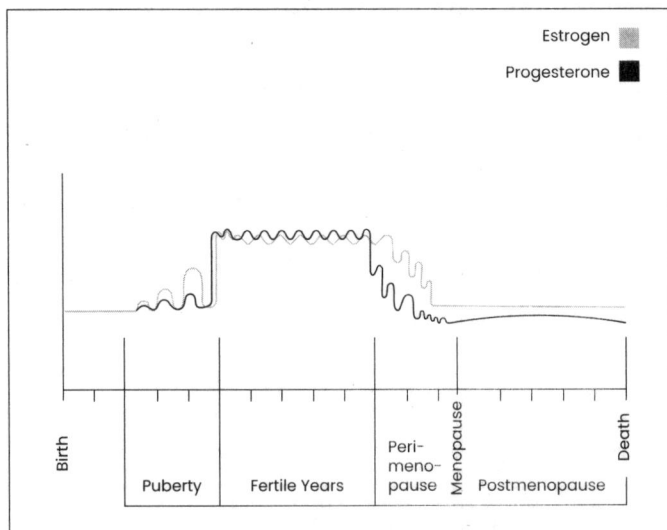

Myth: *My Mental Health Is Destined to Take a Dip*

It is true that about 40 percent of women experience mood-related symptoms during perimenopause, which may include irritability, an uptick in anxious thoughts, rage, weepiness, or feeling blue or lethargic. And many studies suggest that the risk of depression or depressive symptoms increases during perimenopause. It's important to note that there's a difference between having *symptoms* of anxiety and depression and carrying a *diagnosis* of anxiety and depression. Diagnoses are made when symptoms become persistent or daily versus sporadic and cyclic.

Because we know that women's mental health becomes a little more vulnerable during this season, it's a great time to be more proactive about the things that we know benefit mental health—things like journaling, exercising, seeking therapy, meditating, pursuing hobbies, and connecting with friends can make a big difference. (I'll cover more specific strategies in chapters 6 and 9.) Part of the lesson of perimenopause is that it's so important for us to care for ourselves. I know that may feel easier said than done, especially because the perimenopausal years are also typically the time when we're parenting, working, and caring for aging parents. We're busier than ever, but that means we also have all the more reason to prioritize our own well-being. You know the airline oxygen mask saying, so I won't even say it.

Myth: *Perimenopause Is Just Destined to Suck*

It's true that your body is going through epic hormonal changes that have cascading effects, and that these effects can produce symptoms that range from barely noticeable to downright awful. But not everyone has a hard time with perimenopause (although, since you're reading this book, I'm guessing that you're experiencing some challenges!). And if it does turn out to be challenging, it's most definitely not something that you just have to muddle through and wait for it to end. There are so many treatments and things you can do to bring back your quality of life and feel like yourself again—enough to fill an entire book.

The most dangerous thing about this myth is that it can convince you there's nothing you can do to make it better, and not only is that not true, but it's downright dangerous. You deserve to feel better, and you deserve to enjoy strong foundations of health throughout your life, no matter your hormonal status.

Myth: *Weight Gain Is Inevitable*

There is some truth to this, as estrogen helps your body clear glucose from the bloodstream and keep insulin in check, which means perimenopause can change your overall metabolism, but it's very complex.

That's why you can be eating and exercising exactly the same as you did before perimenopause and still gain weight, and also why it can feel like eating less and exercising more doesn't make a dent in those pounds.

There are strategies that serve to help keep your weight in a healthy range—even if that weight is a little higher than it used to be. I'll cover them in chapter 8. In my clinical experience, once women's hormones stabilize as they enter menopause, their body adjusts to its new metabolism and it gets easier to shed a few pounds (and more importantly, build muscle) if that's something they're interested in. But I also am a strong advocate of feeling grateful and loving toward our bodies as they move through this monumental transition. Our bodies may not look like they did when we were twenty years old, but would you really want to be twenty again?

Myth: *Hormone Replacement Therapy Is Unsafe*

The main reason many women and doctors think treating perimenopausal and menopausal symptoms with hormone therapy (HT) is risky is due to a now-infamous study called the Women's Health Initiative (WHI). Before I tell you what the study found, I want to take you back to the 1980s and 1990s, when the majority of menopausal women were given hormone therapy in the form of conjugated equine estrogen (CEE, often sold under the brand name Premarin). At that time, prospective studies found that women who started HT shortly after menopause were living longer with fewer symptoms, had less heart disease, and had stronger bones. In 1992, the American College of Physicians advocated strongly for the use of HT for almost all menopausal women at their annual meeting. Sounds good, right? Okay, let's keep going.

Eager to verify these findings, the National Institutes of Health (NIH) designed the WHI to be a double-blind randomized controlled trial, which is considered to be the gold standard of scientific research because it compares subjects who are given an intervention to a control group who are given a placebo, and neither the researchers nor the subjects know which group is which (removing the risk of confirmation bias, or the tendency of humans to prioritize evidence that proves what they already suspect to be true).

The WHI was designed to have four groups—one group of women who did not have a uterus who took oral CEE only; another group of women without a uterus who took a CEE-only placebo; a third group of women with a uterus and ovaries who took oral Prempro—a combination of CEE and a synthetic form of progesterone called medroxyprogesterone acetate (MPA); and a fourth group with a uterus and ovaries who took an estrogen-progesterone placebo. (These formulations are very important to note, for reasons that will become clear in just a moment.)

The study began in 1993 and was intended to go for ten years. It was very exciting, because the medical community hoped that it would show that HT reduced the risk of heart disease and other chronic diseases. Also important to note is that the WHI was not designed to look at treating menopausal symptoms. In fact, if your symptoms were severe, you were excluded from participating. Another interesting aspect is that the average age of the women enrolled in the studies was mid-sixties. Keep that in mind.

What happened next is that in 2002, the WHI study ended early, reportedly because the safety threshold for breast cancer had been crossed. The media reported that hormone therapy was found to cause a 26 percent increased risk in invasive breast cancer, and everyone—women and doctors alike—threw their hormones and hormone prescriptions in the trash, and the idea that estrogen is dangerous and harmful became deeply rooted in the public psyche. We are still dealing with the fallout today.

In actuality, there was only one arm of the study that saw an increase in breast cancer—the Prempro arm. The increase of risk in this group rose to 2.94 percent, compared to the risk of 2.33 percent in the general population. Technically, the difference between those two numbers is 26 percent, but it is 26 percent of a very small number. Also, it was an increase in the relative risk, which means a comparison between two groups of people—in this case, the women in the Prempro arm versus the general population of women of a similar age. What's more important to consider is the increase in absolute risk, which is the risk of these women developing breast cancer at all. When translated into absolute risk, it means an additional eight women out of ten thousand would develop breast cancer over the course of five years on the oral Prempro when compared to the general population—not the one in four women you might imagine if you heard that 26 percent number on the news.

When they stopped, the WHI researchers also noted an apparent risk of cardiovascular disease and stroke in women in both arms of the study. This, too, scared physicians and the general public and convinced them that HT didn't have any cardiovascular benefits. However, this conclusion was formulated when they were considering all women of all ages in one group.

Now, more than two decades later, researchers have looked more closely at all the data the study gathered. Post hoc analyses have a different story to tell—one that shows how safe HT is and how many benefits it has. For example, in 2007 the WHI researchers reevaluated how the age of the women when they started HT affected outcomes.[2] They found that if you were within ten years of menopause when you started HT, you didn't have bad cardiovascular outcomes. In fact, you had a lower risk of developing diabetes and cardiovascular disease, as well as a greater improvement in symptoms than women in both arms of placebo. That was our first clue that the age at which a woman started HT mattered.

We've also found that formulation and method of delivery really matter. The hormones used in WHI were not chemically identical to natural hormones, which means that they can have unintended effects on your physiology. While Premarin and Prempro are still FDA-approved and available for prescription, we primarily prescribe FDA-approved estradiol and micronized progesterone now, which work more similarly to the hormones our bodies make. In addition, the WHI administered its estrogen orally, in pill form. We now know that when estrogen is taken orally, it has to be processed by the liver; during the metabolization process the liver can produce chemicals that increase the risk of blood clots. So now we more commonly administer estradiol transdermally, via a patch, gel, or a spray, which bypasses the liver and enters directly into the bloodstream, so there are no risks of increased blood clots above a woman's baseline risk.[3]

Let's circle back to the formulation of the hormones. In women who took CEE alone, there was no increased risk of breast cancer, so we have hypothesized that perhaps the synthetic progesterone present in Prempro was problematic. We've since evaluated the risk of different formulations of progesterone, particularly the bioidentical form of progesterone called Prometrium (also known as micronized natural progesterone), which is now widely prescribed, and the great news is that numerous studies have found no increased risk of breast cancer above a woman's baseline.[4] This is a game changer for women who are apprehensive about taking HT due to the risk of breast cancer.

Also, there was good news in the original WHI findings that wasn't reported as widely as the increase in breast cancer risk in the Prempro arm. Years after the WHI closed, the group of women who took estrogen saw only a statistically significant *reduction* in breast cancer risk. And women who took either CEE alone or Prempro, and who went on to be diagnosed with breast cancer, outlived women in the placebo group who were diagnosed with breast cancer.[5] This really puts a new spin on the contextual risks of hormone therapy compared to the immense benefits it delivers.

If you are concerned about a possible link between hormone therapy and breast cancer, your concerns are valid. I also believe that all women deserve the unbiased facts so they can make the best decision for themselves. To give further context to the WHI findings, many women take similar risks on a daily basis—for example, drinking alcohol every day increases relative risk of getting breast cancer by anywhere between 11 and 55 percent, depending on how many drinks you have.[6]

The WHI also didn't factor in the effectiveness of HT to reduce the very bothersome symptoms of menopause, or the long-term benefits of HT, making it impossible at the time to use their findings to conduct a risk-benefit analysis. And there is no data to support the idea that *not* taking hormone therapy lowers breast cancer risk. I further discuss the use of hormone therapy in women who have a family history of breast cancer on page 46.

Today, the Menopause Society's position is that the benefits of HT outweigh the risks for women with no known contraindications to estrogen and who are younger than sixty or within ten years from their last menstrual period.[7] Hormone therapy is an effective and safe option for the majority of women to drastically improve their quality of life, reduce symptoms, and improve long-term health outcomes. While HT is currently FDA-approved for hot flashes, night sweats, the genitourinary syndrome of menopause, and osteopenia, in my clinical experience of treating thousands of women over the last decade, women also see improvements in cognition, brain fog, mood, joint aches and pains, hair, skin, nails, and more. While HT is certainly not the only option, I want to be sure you are gaining confidence in its safety.

If you are still unsure about hormone therapy, perhaps this comparison can help. There is another form of hormone therapy—exogenous hormones (hormones made outside the body), which change physiology—in other words: birth control. This is often a combination of a synthetic progestin (which stops you from ovulating) and synthetic estrogen to alleviate symptoms of low estrogen, such as PMS, PMDD, and hot flashes. The oral dosages of hormones in birth control are typically much higher than the dosage of hormone therapy used to treat perimenopausal and menopausal symptoms.

If birth control is essentially a form of HT, and deemed safe for pre- and perimenopausal women, and HT uses lower dosages of hormones than birth control, then why would using HT be riskier than birth control? If as a society we are not worried about prescribing and or using birth control, we also don't need to have a collective concern about HT.

CONTRAINDICATIONS TO HORMONE THERAPY

There are a handful of evidence-based conditions that suggest hormone therapy isn't appropriate, which I've listed below. However, new data is coming out all the time, which means our understanding of absolute contraindications to HT is continuing to evolve. In addition, every patient is an individual with a unique health history, genetic profile, lifestyle, and set of symptoms. I believe every woman has the right to an individualized risk-benefit analysis and shared decision-making with a well-educated clinician.

The contraindications to hormone therapy are:

- Active or recent history of breast cancer.
- Unprovoked blood clot in leg or in lungs, meaning there was no inciting incident such as a long flight, physical trauma, or prolonged immobilization.
- Any unexplained or concerning vaginal bleeding; however, this is pretty common in perimenopause and is more of a concern in postmenopause. If your doctor has any reason to suspect gynecologic cancer, though, that should be assessed before starting on hormone therapy.
- End-stage liver disease (cirrhosis).
- Recent heart attack.

Some things that are NOT contraindications:

- Smoking.
- Migraines.
- Hypertension.
- Diabetes.
- High cholesterol.
- Autoimmune diseases.
- Clotting disorders (so long as you are using transdermal, not oral, estradiol).
- Family history of breast cancer, clots, or heart attack.

That doesn't mean your clinician should outright ignore these factors if you have them in your health history or that they shouldn't be factored into a risk-benefit analysis. But these are what I call "yellow lights," so we should proceed with caution.

Myth: *Bioidentical Hormones Are All-Natural and Not FDA-Approved*

"Bioidentical" has been widely used as a marketing term to imply that a treatment is all-natural, risk-free, and not something you can get from your doctor. In actuality, what bioidentical means is that a manufactured hormone has a very similar chemical structure to the hormone that is produced by your body, and thus has a very similar effect in your body.

Many bioidentical hormones are FDA-approved, including estradiol (a form of estrogen) and Prometrium (or micronized progesterone), both of which are derived from plants in a lab. There is a popular misconception that the only way to obtain bioidentical hormones is to use a compounding pharmacy, which creates prescription formulations that are individualized to a patient's needs and that are generally not FDA-approved, nor covered by insurance. Yet estradiol and Prometrium are available through your regular pharmacy and typically covered by insurance.

Myth: *If I'm in My Forties, or Still Getting My Period, It's Too Soon to Consider Hormone Therapy*

There is no rule that says you must be in menopause before you start hormone therapy. In fact, hormone therapy is a medical option that can be extremely helpful in supporting women at any time during which their hormones are lowering, such as women diagnosed with premenstrual dysphoric disorder (PMDD, which is essentially PMS on steroids), or who are postpartum, when hormones can drop quickly and contribute to symptoms including insomnia and postpartum depression.

The main reason to consider starting hormone therapy in perimenopause is your symptoms. Remember, perimenopause can last up to ten years. That's a long time. If you are having relentless or increasing symptoms, that means they're likely to persist through most of the perimenopause transition. There's no reason to suffer.

In addition to reducing symptoms, another benefit of starting hormone therapy is that it can be diagnostic. Meaning, if you are experiencing a symptom that resolves after you try hormone therapy—whether it's mood, or a frozen shoulder, or insomnia—you and your clinician will feel much more confident that the symptom was related to the low hormones. And if they don't resolve, you'll know there's another medical reason to keep searching for.

It's also a chance to determine which hormones are triggering which symptoms. For example, if you start adding in an estrogen gel the week before your period and it helps with hot flashes and irritability but not sleep, you and your clinician might next add in progesterone and see if it has an impact. This all helps you better understand your body, and it's my hope that as you go through part II, you'll be able to piece together which hormones often lead to which symptoms and understand how to best tackle each set of your perimenopause symptoms.

Starting hormone therapy in perimenopause also gives you a chance to determine what form, dose, and timing works best for you without waiting until you're in panic mode and in dire need of relief. You'll be more in tune to what your body needs to feel its best, and then, ultimately, you're going to sail into menopause and make that transition a whole lot easier.

We don't have studies that show definitively that starting hormone therapy earlier in perimenopause gives you more long-term benefits, but we suspect it does, based on the fact that women who start earlier on hormone therapy do see long-term benefits, including reductions in cardiovascular disease, less osteopenia and fewer osteoporotic fractures, longer lifespans, and less diabetes.[8] Ongoing research is also highly suggestive that hormone therapy may help support our overall brain health.[9] We can extrapolate that it makes sense to assume that if you start hormone therapy earlier, you may start to accumulate those benefits as well, but more research in this area is needed.

Myth: *If I Have a Personal or Family History of Breast Cancer, It's Unsafe for Me to Take HT*

A family history of breast cancer does not preclude you from taking hormone therapy, because your individual risk of developing breast cancer is influenced much more strongly by your environment than your genetics. Even if you have a genetic mutation that increases your breast cancer risk, but you don't have cancer, HT isn't out of the question—after all, your body has made estrogen for decades without you getting cancer. The general consensus is that bioidentical, FDA-approved estrogen does not increase breast cancer risk above the risk that everyone alive already has, although this is still a complex and individualized decision to be made with your health-care practitioner.

If you are a breast cancer survivor, HT is not an automatic no. Deciding if you're a good candidate or not involves having an in-depth conversation with your clinician, factoring in your risk of recurrence, the type and stage of cancer you had, and what your treatment was, and balancing all that with your quality of life and how significantly your perimenopause symptoms are impacting you. We need more data, and more research is being done every year.

If hormone therapy does not make sense for you from a risk-analysis perspective, there are also some nonhormonal options for addressing perimenopausal symptoms, which I cover in chapter 7.

Myth: *My Vagina Will Never Be the Same*

While it is true that declining estrogen has a significant and most often noticeable impact on the tissues of the genitourinary tract (particularly the labia, vulva, clitoris, vagina, cervix, urethra, ureters, and bladder), it is a widespread myth that women's vaginas are doomed to become dried-up vestiges of their former selves.

Typical changes that may begin in perimenopause and tend to grow more prevalent over time include a loss of lubrication, thinning of the vaginal walls, and a loss of flexibility in the tissues that make up the opening of the vagina—all of which can lead to painful sex—as well as a change in the pH level of the vagina from a more acid pH, around 5, to a more alkaline pH, at 6 or 7, which can pave the way for increased urinary tract infections. You may also start to get inconclusive or abnormal results on your pap smear as a result of the general atrophy of the tissues.

Now for the good part: Vaginal estrogen, which comes in the form of creams, suppositories, or rings, can reverse these otherwise-unavoidable changes. Vaginal estrogen is local, meaning the estrogen stays in the vaginal tissues and doesn't get absorbed into the bloodstream and travel throughout the body, which in turn means there are no known risks of vaginal estrogen. Many studies have established that it is safe for all women, including breast cancer survivors.[10]

Vaginal estrogen works. It helps to improve lubrication, which means more comfortable sex as well as improved vaginal health. It also works to restore blood flow, sensitivity, and resilience to the tissues, which means more pleasure, better orgasms, and fewer UTIs. It also reduces the pH level to its more preferred level, which is what helps all the cells function at their best. It really is the gold standard for pelvic floor and vaginal health.

For all these reasons, I wish that vaginal estrogen were available over the counter. We put hyaluronic acid and retinol on our facial skin every night, so we should be giving the labia and lower pelvic floor tissues the TLC they need. Unfortunately, not only does this type of estrogen require a prescription, but there is currently a very scary-sounding black box label on vaginal estrogen products. The FDA requires this label, even though vaginal estrogen does not carry the same risks as systemic estrogen, which is used to treat all the other symptoms of menopause. There are many clinicians and advocates doing the hard work of appealing to the FDA to remove this misleading warning, and I wholeheartedly support their efforts. Because the more access women have to vaginal estrogen, the better the quality of life will be for all women at midlife and beyond.

One important point: While vaginal estrogen can do a lot of wonderful things, reducing hot flashes isn't one of them. Since vaginal estrogen doesn't travel throughout the body via the bloodstream, it doesn't help address any symptoms of estrogen loss that occur beyond the genitourinary tract.

Myth: *If You're on Systemic Hormone Therapy, You Shouldn't Add Vaginal Estrogen*

Forty percent of women on systemic hormone therapy still need to use local vaginal estrogen in order to relieve their genitourinary symptoms. That's because these tissues have the most estrogen receptors of anywhere in the body, and sometimes they just need some extra TLC.

IF YOU DO ONE THING: BEGIN LOGGING YOUR SYMPTOMS

Now that you know what's fact and what's fiction when it comes to perimenopause, it's time to turn your attention to what's going on with *you*.

Even though perimenopause is a universal experience for women, we'll all experience it a bit differently. This means no two women are going to have the exact same treatment plan.

The way to personalize your path is to start tracking your symptoms. In the same place you are tracking the start and end dates of your periods (which was your quick assignment at the end of chapter 1—you are doing this, yes?), start writing down the date and any out-of-the-ordinary symptoms you experienced that day.

If you had a headache, bad gas, crazy dreams, a short fuse, spotting, or you blew through several super-maxi pads, write it down. Do this every day, or catch up on a couple of days at a time if you forget. Put a star next to the symptoms that really disrupted your day.

This list, especially the starred items, is going to help you prioritize what set of symptoms you want to address first, because it will be easy to see which ones are the most disruptive. And when you cross-reference the symptoms you're experiencing with where you are in your cycle (because you've been tracking those start and end dates), you'll also be able to see which symptoms are happening cyclically. This list is also going to help your clinician piece together what is going on with your hormones and your body and work with you to develop a treatment plan you can feel confident about.

CHAPTER 3

Assess Your Symptoms; Set Your Priorities

A typical pattern I see among my patients: They are inspired to book an appointment with me because they are not sleeping. Maybe night sweats are keeping them up, or maybe they can't shut off their busy brains, or both. Either way, they struggle with getting to sleep or staying asleep, or both, which is making them irritable. They're yelling at their partner, their kids, drivers of the cars ahead of them on the road, maybe even their colleagues. And they've gained weight that they can't seem to shed, even though they haven't changed their diet or exercise habits. Taken together, it's making them feel a little crazy, and rightfully so.

After going through the very same process with them that I'll walk you through in this chapter, we identify the symptoms that are plaguing them the most and start there. Very often, the top priorities are dealing with the sleeplessness, crankiness, and brain fog. A standard regimen might include a prescription for oral progesterone, taken about an hour before bed. Because progesterone is calming, it can help you not fall prey to swirling thoughts that can keep you up and also help you stay sleepy through the night (so if you wake up to go to the bathroom, you hopefully can get back to sleep).

We would likely also discuss swapping out sweetened coffee drinks or sugary foods they've been using to boost their energy for something higher in protein and fiber, like nuts or an apple with peanut butter, so that they are less likely to experience a post-sugar crash.

After a few weeks, when their sleep is noticeably better—most women still have some tough nights, but for the most part, they're getting a good seven hours a night—they now have the energy to add in some exercise, which further helps with irritability (because it relieves stress); sleep (because it tires you out); and weight gain (because it boosts metabolism). In four to six months, they feel so much better that they can't even remember just how poorly they were feeling when they first came to see me.

While your symptoms may be different from the ones I used in this example—after all, as we'll cover in this chapter, there are dozens of different perimenopausal symptoms—the process of remedying your group of symptoms is exactly the same. You have to get clear on what your symptoms are, identify which ones you want to target, decide (ideally with a clinician you trust) what treatments and tools to try, give yourself a chance to experience the results, and then repeat the process until you've got your quality of life back.

It sounds simple, and for the most part, it is. But it's not always easy—when your symptoms are making you miserable and worried, it's hard to have clarity on what you should do. In this chapter, we'll create that clarity. First, you'll learn how the many symptoms of perimenopause cluster into what I call *symptom sets*. Experiencing multiple symptoms of perimenopause at one time can be a bummer, but also helpful, because you can avoid the confusion of addressing each symptom individually. Doing so is often why it takes women up to seven appointments with different clinicians and specialists before they tie their symptoms to perimenopause and receive a treatment plan that addresses the root of their symptoms. Once you figure out which symptom set you're experiencing, you can address multiple issues with just a few well-chosen interventions.

If going through this process makes you realize you are dealing with multiple symptom sets—as most of my patients are—know that for each intervention you try, you tend to free up more energy and bandwidth to help you get to the bottom of your next symptom set. To use a financial analogy, addressing your perimenopausal symptom sets is like getting compound interest. The more you put in at the beginning of the process, and the more consistent you are over time, the more exponentially those benefits will grow. In this case, instead of compounding money, you compound vitality and well-being, and the confidence and ease that come from knowing you're setting yourself up for better health over the rest of your life.

In this chapter, I'll walk you through some questions (the same questions I ask each of my patients) to help you get a clear view of how perimenopause may or may not be affecting your life, identify your most disruptive symptom set, and set your priorities for which group of symptoms you want to target first.

Answering these questions *does* require a fair amount of self-reflection, but it's a vital step because perimenopause is not a one-size-fits all journey, and self-knowledge is critical for charting your path and finding the approaches that will work for you. Anytime you feel resistance to taking the time to think through your answers, just remind yourself of the returns you'll experience now (fewer symptoms, higher quality of life) and the dividends (better long-term health, stronger bones, lower risk of heart disease and dementia) you'll reap later. But first, let's take a look at what the symptoms of perimenopause are, so that you can collect all the data you need to do a full assessment of your own personal array of symptoms.

The Thirty-Four Symptoms of Perimenopause

Welcome to the smorgasbord of symptoms that your changing hormones can create. As you read through these, make sure each one you're experiencing is on the list you started at the end of chapter 2 (it's possible you've been feeling some things on this list but didn't write them down because you didn't realize that they could be related to perimenopause).

I understand that seeing these all gathered in one place can be overwhelming, even maddening—why does perimenopause have to be so intense?! Keep in mind that we are going to address how to lessen these symptoms in the coming chapters.

1. **Acne.** As your ratio of testosterone to estrogen changes (because estrogen is declining) it can promote acne, as well as hair growing in new places (like your chin).

2. **Allergies.** Fluctuating hormone levels can cause spikes in histamine, the chemical that triggers allergic reactions as part of your body's immune response.

3. **Anxiety.** Declining progesterone, which is calming, and estrogen, which boosts serotonin, can inspire an uptick in anxious thoughts—sometimes significantly so.

4. **Bloating.** As estrogen declines, the bacterial population in your gut shifts, making digestion a little slower and promoting the formation of gas, which can make you feel bloated.

5. **Body odor.** If you think you've been smelling differently lately, you're probably not wrong. This is because the same rise in testosterone relative to estrogen can foster the growth of odor-causing bacteria in your sweat.[1]

6. **Brain fog.** The Study of Women's Health Across the Nation (SWAN) found that women going through their menopause transition experienced a decline in cognitive performance—primarily in their ability to learn new things. Thankfully, they also found that this dip is temporary, with performance rebounding to premenopausal levels once they got past menopause.[2]

7. **Breast tenderness.** This is often one of the first symptoms of perimenopause, but it is also often the first to resolve. It generally occurs when estrogen is high and progesterone is low. And in early perimenopause especially, estrogen can spike, while progesterone slowly declines.

8. **Brittle nails.** Estrogen supports the production of two key factors in nail health—keratin and collagen. As it declines, so can the strength of your nails.

9. **Changes in taste and dry mouth.** Even your mouth contains estrogen receptors, and as it declines you may produce less saliva, which then can lead to dry mouth, a burning sensation, or even

numbness on your tongue. It can also create a welcoming environment to harmful bacteria and lead to changes in your dental health. Many patients also tell me that food tastes different, too, because saliva plays a key role in breaking down food and with less of it, all the flavors of food may be less accessible.

10. **Changes in sense of smell.** Taste and smell are closely linked, and the mucous membranes in the nose become drier as estrogen goes down, which can impact your sense of smell. Maybe perfumes you used to like now smell off, or you can't tolerate strong smells that once didn't bother you.

11. **Changes in hair.** The decline in collagen and keratin can impact your hair, too, making it more prone to breakage or changing its texture. Many women notice that their hair starts thinning in perimenopause, too (myself included). Declining estrogen can actually shrink your hair follicles, which slows down growth and promotes shedding.

12. **Decreased libido.** A waning—or completely absent—interest in having sex is very common. One study that followed Australian women over eight years found that 42 percent of who were in early perimenopause reported some level of sexual dysfunction at the start of the study. After eight years had passed, that more than doubled to 88 percent.[3] Changing genital tissues can make sex painful, lack of sleep can make you feel too tired, depressive symptoms can make you less interested in pleasure, and dropping testosterone can stymie desire.

13. **Difficulty experiencing pleasure.** Both the mental and the physical changes of perimenopause can leave you feeling like your internal mood meter is stuck on "blah." Depression-like symptoms affect about 40 percent of perimenopausal women.[4]

14. **Dizzy spells.** There are a lot of ways declining estrogen can contribute to dizziness—changes in the inner ear (where balance is regulated), fatigue, heart palpitations, and anxiety are all more common now as a result, and each of these factors can lead

to dizziness. Research has found that dizziness occurs in up to 35 percent of women.[5]

15. **Electric shock sensations.** Estrogen helps to regulate the nervous system; as it gets more erratic so can nerve function, meaning you may experience what some of my patients call "zingers," tingling sensations down your arms or legs.

16. **Fatigue.** This can be a direct result of interrupted sleep; it can also occur because of the decline in hormones, which, from an evolutionary perspective, help give you the energy to be primed and ready to get out there and mate, reproduce, and care for offspring.

17. **Headaches/migraines.** Women are more prone to headaches, including migraines, than men throughout their lives, but the prevalence of migraines peaks for women in their late thirties, which is when hormones can start their perimenopausal shifting.[6]

18. **Heavy bleeding.** Progesterone is the orchestrator of your uterine lining. When it starts diminishing, things can go a little haywire. (Although there are also other, nonhormonal reasons for heavy bleeding—refer to chapter 4 for more information if this is something you're dealing with.)

19. **Hot flashes.** The brain has receptors for estrogen, including in the hypothalamus, which regulates changes in body temperature. When estrogen declines, the hypothalamus can go rogue, making it harder for your inner thermostat to accommodate even the smallest of shifts in ambient temperature. Up to half of perimenopausal women experience hot flashes.[7]

20. **Incontinence.** Lots of factors contribute to this indignity, including a decline in integrity of the tissues in the bladder, urinary tract, and pelvic floor. Most often, this is stress incontinence, meaning, it happens when you sneeze, cough, or jump. But your bladder can also get overactive (more frequent urges to go), or your bladder and pelvic floor muscles may get weak so that urine leaks out. Incontinence affects 30 to 40 percent of women at midlife, and becomes more common as you get older.[8]

21. **Irregular heartbeat/heart palpitations.** Estrogen helps keep the different chambers of your heart in sync, so as it becomes volatile, so can your heartbeat. Also, an increase in anxiety can also increase heart rate (and an increase in heart rate can spike anxiety).

22. **Irregular periods.** This is often the first sign of perimenopause. Your periods often start coming more frequently (although they could also be further apart), or you skip a period, or your flow starts getting heavier or more erratic, before eventually spacing out in later perimenopause.

23. **Irritability.** Declining estrogen can definitely shorten your fuse. Just as you may have felt testy during PMS (the phase of your cycle when estrogen is the lowest), you may now be feeling it even more acutely as estrogen's dips go even lower. Many of my patients tell me they're beyond irritable—they're rageful. It's all within the realm of normalcy. (Meaning, you are not a bad person!)

24. **Itchy/dry skin.** In general, declining estrogen equals dryness, because estrogen promotes elasticity and moisture, and this includes in your skin (the largest organ in the body). If you've been noticing drier, itchier skin, you're not imagining it.

25. **Joint pain and muscle aches.** Since estrogen is anti-inflammatory, it's like you gradually lose access to your innate version of ibuprofen. It often manifests as low back pain or a frozen shoulder. We now call these changes the muscoloskeletal syndrome of menopause and yes, it often starts in perimenopause.

26. **Mood changes.** In addition to irritability and rage, you may also find yourself feeling more anxious (generally due to declining progesterone) or more blue (generally due to declining estrogen and as a result, serotonin).

27. **Night sweats.** These are hot flashes that happen in the middle of the night. You can blame lower estrogen levels.

28. **Panic attacks.** An increase in anxiety and heart palpitations can add up to full-blown panic attacks. And some hot flashes can be

intense, especially if you don't yet realize that is what's happening to you, which may cause so much worry that it turns into a panic attack. Interestingly, research has found that women who suffer from frequent panic attacks in perimenopause have a different population of gut bacteria than women who don't, highlighting how these symptoms are often intertwined with one another.[9]

29. **Sleep disturbances.** Of all the symptoms of perimenopause, this may be one of the most brutal, because sleeping poorly has such wide-ranging negative effects on mood, energy, mental clarity, and metabolism. Research shows that nearly 40 percent of perimenopausal women have sleep problems.[10]

30. **Skin changes.** As you enter perimenopause, you lose up to 5 percent of your collagen production each year, which can contribute to declining elasticity and the appearance of aging skin. Skin is also drier now, thanks to declining estrogen, and you may notice more age spots, that wounds take a little longer to heal, and that your skin is getting thinner.

31. **Tinnitus, or ringing in the ears.** The lack of estrogen can dry out your ear canals, too, making the tissues in there more vulnerable to wear and tear, including in the cells that turn sound waves into electrical signals to your brain.

32. **More frequent UTIs.** As the tissues in your urinary tract lose some of their resilience, and the pH of the bladder and urethra increases due to the loss of estrogen, unfriendly bacteria have an easier time taking root, making you more susceptible to urinary tract infections.

33. **Vaginal dryness.** This is a hallmark of perimenopause, because the vagina has the highest concentration of estrogen (and androgen) receptors. When they decline, you produce less moisture and mucus, which can lead to painful sex and a change in the pH of the vagina, which then further contributes to dryness.

34. **Weight gain.** Estrogen affects the way your body regulates glucose and insulin in a complex manner. Since insulin is a fat-storage

hormone, this can result in extra weight accumulating, typically in the belly, even though you haven't been eating more or changed the way you eat.

Grouping Your Symptoms into a Set

If you are looking at how many symptoms you've experienced and feeling daunted because the list is long, grouping them into a set makes them more manageable.

Perimenopausal symptoms tend to cluster because they often share a common root, such as a particular declining hormone. By grouping your symptoms and targeting the root they all share, you can remedy a lot of them at once. I've grouped the symptoms into the most common clusters that I see in my patients. Seeing how some seemingly unrelated things fit together into a set can make the process of feeling better less overwhelming.

Here's a brief overview of each of the symptom sets:

- *Bleeding 'til you drop*—more frequent, more intense periods with a flow that can look like a crime scene. Heavy bleeding often is related to anatomical factors—such as uterine polyps, fibroids, multiple pregnancies, endometriosis, or adenomyosis. It can also be related simply to the decline in both progesterone, which regulates menstrual flow, and estrogen.
- *Lying awake and worrying*—insomnia, anxiety, and even heart palpitations that seem to come from nowhere. This cluster of symptoms tends to stem from a decline in progesterone, which typically starts sooner than the decline in estrogen.
- *Dragging yourself through life*—fatigue, difficulty experiencing pleasure, feeling blue, joint pain. These symptoms are typically related to the lowering of estrogen.
- *Feeling unrecognizable to yourself*—hot flashes, dry skin, seemingly visible aging, irritability, brain fog. Typically, we can thank the

decline of the trifecta—estrogen, progesterone, and testosterone—for this cluster of symptoms.

- *Gaining weight for no (apparent) reason*—You can't button your jeans suddenly—even though your diet hasn't changed. This is a downstream effect of a decline in estrogen, which can trigger changes in insulin sensitivity, hormones that control appetite, where you store fat, and a rise in cortisol.

- *The silent symptoms*—these include the cardiovascular, bone, and brain changes that happen as our hormones recede. I call them "silent" because you don't notice your bones changing or your cholesterol rising. But they are happening sooner or later—maybe not right at this moment if you are in the early stages of perimenopause—but they are menopause's close companions. Every woman will experience these symptoms to some degree. Don't panic, though—not only will I walk you through these risks, but I'll also tell you how to reduce them.

If you are reading through these and thinking, *Oh no, I have more than one symptom set*, that is totally normal. You may even feel like you are experiencing all of the symptom sets. It is possible to treat multiple symptom sets, but not all at once, because you want to be able to evaluate how effective each remedy is before you try another, and you can't do that accurately if you're trying a bunch of different things all at the same time. For now, you need to prioritize. And thinking through all of this and writing down your answers to the questions I'm about to ask you is how you'll do that.

Charting Your Course

It's time to get out that notebook or journal or open your Notes app or a Google doc so you can start to clearly see what's been happening with you and where you want to go from here.

I know you may not want to take the time to think about what's been going on with you. How do I know? Because whenever I'm reading a book that tells me to get out a notebook, journal, or legal pad, I'll admit that I think, *Oh, hell no! I'm reading; isn't that enough?* Trust me, I understand that desire to just get to the information, already. Yet here I go, asking you to do the very same thing. Here's why:

One of the most upsetting things about perimenopause is how confusing it can be. You may feel like you might be losing your mind, or like you are making up symptoms in your head, or you may even wonder if you're starting to exaggerate what's not really that big of a deal. These feelings can then keep you from seeking out ways to alleviate those symptoms.

Remember that perimenopause can easily last as long as ten years. It's too long to wait to feel better (and there are no guarantees that menopause will be substantially better). Also, there are hormone-related changes happening to your bones, brain, heart, and metabolism, and the longer you wait to address them, the more ground you may have lost.

Taking an objective look at everything you've been experiencing helps you know that you haven't been imagining things. It increases your self-awareness and your self-knowledge. This also helps you prioritize your next steps, which is absolutely vital. By targeting your most bothersome symptoms, you'll get a more efficient treatment plan and start to feel better faster. Otherwise, you're just throwing spaghetti at the wall.

This is a time to think about *you*, and what health and happiness mean to you. How you treat your body during perimenopause absolutely sets the stage for the next three to four decades. Taking positive steps now puts you on a trajectory toward happiness and good health, instead of leaving you to struggle through the aging process, wishing you had done things differently.

Question 1: When did these symptoms start?

Review the list of symptoms you've created—and hopefully updated now that you've learned the thirty-four most common perimenopause symptoms. Your answers to this question can help tease out how far along you might be into your perimenopausal transition. They can also give clarity and validate your own experience—it's much harder to dismiss something you've noted in your own handwriting than a thought. It will also help your clinician get a full picture of what's going on with you. And finally, your answer will also provide a "before" snapshot, so in a few weeks or months you can look back and be amazed at how far you've come.

Question 2: *If you get periods (skip this if you don't get periods right now), how are your symptoms related to your cycle?*
This will help you get a better understanding of which hormones are being affected and help you feel prepared in knowing when you might have some rough days ahead that you can better plan for.

Question 3: *How are symptoms affecting your job? Your personal relationships? Your mental health?*
Don't hold back here, because quality of life is *so* important. Your answers to this multipart question might motivate you to try something new, and they also will help demonstrate to your clinician how important it is that they help you find an effective treatment plan.

Question 4: *If you had a magic wand and could make one of your symptoms immediately disappear, what would it be?*
This question is all about helping you prioritize the symptom set that's giving you the most trouble, so you know exactly where to put your energy first.

Question 5: *What would the second symptom you'd target be? The third?*
In my experience, there's rarely just one symptom that's chipping away at your quality of life. Answering this question—both parts—helps create a road map that extends further than just the first step.

Question 6: *Imagine it is three to six months from now and you are your healthiest, happiest self. What are you doing to maintain that feeling? (For example, are you back to your morning run? Cooking dinner again? Going back to your book club? Creating your art?)*

When you're not feeling well, it can be hard to remember what feeling good is like. Your answer to this question can help motivate you. It can also capture what your inner knowing and intuition have to say about what's going to help you. You're not committing to doing all of these things every day, but since you know a lot already about what helps you feel good, this is your chance to list those things in one place.

Question 7: *What have you already tried, and did these things help, or not?*

This is validating on multiple levels—by allowing you to give yourself credit for the effort you've put in, by helping you clearly see what has helped and what hasn't, and by allowing you to decide what things you'll keep doing as you move forward and what you can let go.

Question 8: *Do you have an idea of what would help you at this point?*

This is a great way to capture the treatments and tactics you've been contemplating or are seeing flash by in your social media feed. Sharing your answer to this question with your clinician also helps them to meet you where you are by suggesting treatments that you are open to.

Question 9: *What's going on in your life—with your kids, pets, partner, job, and parents? Did you just change jobs? Are you going through a divorce? Starting a new relationship?*

These answers can affect your current capacity for change. After all, a treatment option has to fit into your life and lifestyle. If you're traveling a lot, or taking care of a sick parent, you need to factor that in and make your plans more realistic and consistent for you.

Where to Go from Here

The next part of this book is a bit of a choose-your-own adventure. I suggest looking at your answer to question 4—the first symptom you'd make go away if you had a magic wand—and then flipping to the chapter that addresses that symptom set. After all, this is your most troublesome symptom. Let's get this trending in a better direction. I want you to get relief as soon as possible!

My only caution here is that if heavy and irregular bleeding is your top symptom, you definitely want to tackle that first, as some of the treatments for other symptom sets—namely, hormone therapy—can make this worse.

From there, I advise you, just as I advise my patients, to follow the 75 percent rule: Stick with one symptom set until you feel that this area is about 75 percent improved. It doesn't need to be perfect, or like it was when you were twenty-two, but improved to where you're feeling pretty good. Then, you're ready to tackle the symptom set that you listed in question 5, where you listed the second and third symptoms that you'd wish away using your magic wand.

I'm not suggesting you skip any symptom set chapters that don't apply to you. All your hormones will change at different rates and at different times, so while one symptom set doesn't apply to you today, it could two years from now. (Remember, perimenopause is long!) And even if you don't have, say, heavy bleeding, your sister or friend might, and reading through that chapter will help you help her.

But for now, skip ahead to the chapter on your most bothersome symptom set and let's start creating and following your personalized road map to feeling better. Before you go, though, let's discuss how to talk to your doctor about your symptoms—because you will want someone who (1) knows about perimenopause; (2) listens to you; and (3) is open to shared decision-making to help you put your full treatment plan into place.

How to Talk to Your Doctor About Perimenopause

My best advice for having a satisfying conversation with your doctor about getting help for your symptoms is to schedule a problem-focused visit—don't try to shoehorn it into your annual exam. At your yearly physical, your doctor has a lot to get through, including updating your health history, going over your medications and possibly prescribing refills or changing doses, determining which immunizations you might need, going over the screenings you may be due for, and determining which blood tests they want you to have. And unfortunately, in a traditional health-care model, all of this needs to fit into a fifteen- or twenty-minute appointment slot. It's just not enough time to have a full conversation about something new.

When you call to make this appointment (or book it in your patient portal), make it clear that you want to discuss perimenopause—let's start putting it on our doctors' radars! You will also want to do some prep for this visit so you can get the most out of it. Trust me on this, preparing ahead of time will hopefully set you up for a more satisfying visit.

- List the symptoms you've been experiencing (even if this list is twenty items long), and for how long.
- Prioritize the top one, two, or three symptoms you want to address first because they are impacting your quality of life the most (for example, you might say, "I really need help with the night sweats the most because they are leading to my daytime fatigue, irritability, and sugar cravings").
- For each symptom, record all the ways it is impacting your quality of life as well as what you've already tried to remedy it. Really get detailed here: If you're not sleeping and it's affecting your performance at work, or if you're irritable and you're fighting with your partner and considering separating, or if you're experiencing painful sex to the point that you're avoiding it and that's leading to self-esteem issues or strain in your relationship, say so.

- Have the start and end dates of your last three to five periods (which you wrote down at the end of chapter 1—right?), and compare that to what your periods were doing when you were premenopausal.

Going in with this information printed out and in hand will help you have the maximum time available for discussion (so you don't have to waste time flipping through your phone or calendar to try to figure out when your last three periods started, for example).

If you'd like to discuss hormone therapy, you can say something like "I've been reading up on the research and I'd like to use shared decision-making to determine what's right for me." You can even bring a copy of this book in with you—dog-ear the pages that relate to your top-priority symptoms. If your conversation leaves you feeling unheard or dismissed, then seek a second opinion.

For a fill-in-the-blank script you can use to organize your thoughts (it's easy to forget what you wanted to say once you're in the examination room!), look in "Appendix C: Fill-in-the-Blank-Script" at the back of this book.

Bringing up your concerns with your doctor helps you to help yourself. It may also inspire your clinician to fill in any gaps in their own knowledge, which has the potential to help a lot more women. A rule of thumb to keep in mind is that a single clinician trained about perimenopause can affect more than a thousand women. In the class I offer for clinicians, the feedback I hear is that they are hungry for this information and eager to implement it in their practices so that more women can find relief for their symptoms. (See "Appendix B: Resources" for a link to that class.)

From my particular stance within the medical community, we likely have at least another five to ten years before the majority of doctors are well-trained in perimenopause. That means that you may well know more about perimenopause and its possible treatments than your doctor does (because you've been doing your research, including reading this book). It can be potentially awkward to have a conversation with a doctor on a topic that they don't (yet) know well, but it might help to realize that you are accelerating the rate of change.

According to research my team and I conducted and presented at the annual meeting of the Menopause Society in 2024, the second-biggest fear women have about hormone therapy (second only to the fear of breast cancer) is that of being dismissed by their doctors. There's a gap between the level of women's interest in hormone therapy—which is skyrocketing—and their confidence in being prepared to have an informed conversation with their doctors—but it is slowly creeping up.

If you've done all the things I've just outlined and you still don't feel like your clinician adequately addressed your concerns, it's time for a second opinion. Luckily, you have more options for seeking out that second opinion every day. I've listed multiple places to search for a clinician who has been certified in menopausal medicine in "Appendix B: Resources" section of this book.

Now that you have your priorities set, and you know how to partner with your doctor to support you through this process, it's time to turn to the chapter covering your most troublesome symptom set. (I'll trust that you'll read the other chapters in part II as you're ready!)

PINPOINT YOUR PERIMENOPAUSAL SYMPTOM SET

CHAPTER 4

Bleeding 'Til You Drop

Lisa, a forty-three-year-old ninth-grade schoolteacher, starts bleeding during class. She bleeds so much, so quickly, it seeps right through her pants and she has to dig a sweatshirt out of the lost-and-found bin to wrap around her waist—just like some of her students occasionally have to do. What is she, fourteen again?

Lately it seems like she never knows when her period is coming. Once it does finally start, it can last for weeks. She jokes to her friends that it feels like her period is sucking the life right out of her, because lately she has been feeling like every little thing is a huge exertion—climbing the stairs to her bedroom, putting her grocery bags in the back of her car, even picking up her cat. What Lisa doesn't yet realize is that she's become anemic.

She's had several appointments with her gynecologist to look for a reason she might be bleeding so heavily—such as uterine fibroids, endometrial polyps, a bleeding disorder, or uterine cancer (even though uterine cancer most often doesn't occur until after age fifty, doctors will still want to rule it out—see the sidebar on p. 70). But they haven't found anything. Lisa starts to miss work because her periods are so heavy and painful, and she's starting to fantasize about having her uterus removed. Not that she's excited about the thought of surgery, but it would mean the bleeding would stop.

Lisa is by no means alone. Research has found that up to 30 percent of women have what's termed "abnormal uterine bleeding"—although, how abnormal can something be that up to one in three women experience? One of my patients recently quipped, "I thought getting older meant getting your period less!" But the opposite is often true—as your hormones start their perimenopausal fluctuations, the decline in progesterone can lead to increased bleeding—heavier, longer-lasting, and more frequent periods.

Why? Progesterone is the conductor of the uterine lining—it says when to build up, when to release, and when to do nothing while waiting for further clues. Without the conductor's cues, the lining can be like a kid with no parental supervision, going a little crazy simply because it can.

Another hormonal factor is that estrogen levels tend to be really erratic in perimenopause, with higher highs and lower lows than when you were premenopausal. When it spikes, estrogen is basically saying, "Get ready to have a baby" to the uterus, which cues the uterine lining to grow thicker. Even a minor surge in estrogen can have a big effect, because progesterone tends to lower steadily throughout menopause, making a little bit more estrogen exert more of an influence because there is less progesterone to counter it. Double whammy.

This is why I recommend that if you are experiencing heavy bleeding, you seek to treat it first before addressing any other symptom sets— because while adding estrogen can make a wide swath of perimenopause symptoms better, it can potentially make bleeding worse. Better to get your bleeding in an improved place first.

BLEEDING 'TIL YOU DROP AT A GLANCE

Symptoms

- Frequent and/or heavy periods, possibly with heavier than normal clotting
- New onset of cramping
- Fatigue

- Potential symptoms of anemia (refer to sidebar on page 72)
- Possibility of constipation or urinary retention (as anatomical factors could be applying pressure to your colon or bladder)

Causative Factors

- Volatile estrogen and declining progesterone
- Potential anatomical factors such as fibroids, polyps, or endometriosis (see a full list on page 73)

Before we get into remedies, I want to acknowledge just how challenging it is to live with heavy bleeding. It can be painful, as oftentimes when flow is heavy the uterus is contracting, like a mini version of labor, in an effort to expel its lining. And if you have a condition like endometriosis or adenomyosis, the pain level might go well beyond normal menstrual cramps. It's also a lot to manage—changing pads, tampons, menstrual cups, period underwear, or some combination of these multiple times a day, worrying about bleeding through your clothes, doing an extra load of laundry, bringing a change of clothes with you in case it happens. Plus, the costs of menstrual-care products can add up.

Heavy bleeding can impact all aspects of your life. You may feel hesitant to exercise, because who wants to do a downward dog pose or go on a jog when you're nervous about soaking through your tampon, again? Sometimes, working out worsens the bleeding, as exercise increases blood flow throughout the body, including to the uterus (although exercise can also help relax your muscles, including those in your uterus, which can decrease any cramping you may be experiencing). Continued heavy flow can sap your energy, impacting your performance at work, or you might not feel up to socializing with friends. You're less likely to feel like having sex, or being spontaneous.

From a health perspective, repeated heavy bleeding can make you vulnerable to anemia (low iron levels.) As we bleed, we're shedding both accumulated endometrial lining as well as fresh blood cells, which have the vital job of carrying oxygen to all our vital organs and extremities, and when our blood is less oxygenated, that can trigger a wide range of other symptoms (see the following sidebar for a full list).

SYMPTOMS OF ANEMIA

Anemia is easy to treat with iron supplementation, but you first need to confirm via a definitive blood test that you have it, since taking more iron than you need could contribute to inflammation.[1] If you have heavy bleeding and are experiencing two or more of the following symptoms of anemia, give your doctor a call to request blood work.

- Brittle nails
- Chest pain
- Cold hands or feet
- Dizziness or lightheadedness
- Dry skin
- Feeling tired
- Feeling weak
- Headaches
- Irregular heartbeat
- Shortness of breath

Despite all this, as women we are trained to just suck it up and stick it out. We pop Advil and call in sick when it's really bad. Your doctor might suggest heavy bleeding is normal, or they may skip right over perimenopause as a possible cause and start exploring other conditions such as endometriosis, unknown pelvic pain, or even uterine cancer, adding to your anxiety when the most likely explanation is shifting hormones.

Despite the pain, the inconvenience, and the health risks, there is good news: There are multiple evidence-based effective medical treatments that can address the root cause of heavy bleeding and provide relief, as well as multiple ways you can support yourself during this phase of midlife.

Finding the right treatment requires identifying all the reasons why your bleeding might have increased. Whether the cause of your intense periods is shifting hormones, something anatomical, or both, there are multiple ways to treat and support yourself through this symptom set. Take a deep breath and let it all the way out—it is about to get better.

Anatomical Factors That Contribute to Heavy Bleeding

Often, heavy bleeding is the result of a confluence of hormonal changes and anatomical realities such as polyps or fibroids. Both essentially create extra surface area of the uterine lining—meaning there is more tissue available to respond to the hormonal signals (which are already out of whack); and there is more uterine lining, meaning there is more lining to shed, hence the heavier bleeding. These are the most common anatomical factors that may make your bleeding worse.

Polyps are noncancerous growths made out of the endometrial tissue that lines the uterus. They occur in up to 35 percent of females and are most commonly formed in your forties as you approach menopause.[2] Polyps form in a range of sizes—from a few millimeters to a few centimeters—and develop in a lot of places—on the inside of the uterus, on the outside of the uterus, on the cervix, or even in the pelvic wall. If the polyps are on your cervix, they are prone to bleeding because the cervix contains a lot of blood vessels. In perimenopausal women, polyps are very rarely cancerous, although it's still important to get them checked out by your clinician. Uterine polyps are sometimes seen on an ultrasound, while polyps on the cervix may be seen during a routine pelvic exam. Uterine polyps can be removed during a procedure called a dilation and curettage (D&C for short), which is now available as an outpatient procedure done under anesthesia. A clinician dilates the cervix and uses a curette, a spoon-shaped instrument, to remove growths. Cervical polyps can often be removed in a gynecologist's office. Note that polyps don't typically cause pain.

While polyps grow from the wall of the uterus, **fibroids** develop within the muscular uterine wall. Unlike polyps, fibroids are made of dense, fibrous connective tissue, and can grow large enough to press on other organs (such as the rectum or colon) and cause discomfort and constipation. Like polyps, fibroids can grow to varying sizes.

Fibroids are often diagnosed with an ultrasound. If an ultrasound isn't sufficient, your clinician may prefer you to have a sonohysterogram, where a saline solution is introduced into the uterus to give the imaging more of a 3D appearance, like the difference between the regular sonogram and a 3D ultrasound you may have had if you've been pregnant.

Possible treatments include a D&C for smaller fibroids. Bigger fibroids may require a myomectomy, which is surgery that can be done either transvaginally (through the vagina), laparoscopically, or abdominally, depending on the placement and size of your fibroids. If your surgeon is planning a myomectomy, it is common to have either a CT or an MRI scan done beforehand to get the best possible imaging before the fibroid is surgically removed.

Sometimes, fibroids can shrink in size postmenopausally as there is less blood flow to the uterus (due to the declining estrogen levels) and therefore fewer resources, such as oxygen and nutrients, delivered to the fibroids, causing them to naturally shrink in size. But this is not always a guarantee. Postmenopausal women can still have fibroids.

FIBROID SYMPTOMS (IN ADDITION TO HEAVY BLEEDING)

- Distended abdomen (if the fibroid is large).
- Constipation (as a fibroid can press on the bowels).
- Fertility issues (depending on how many fibroids you have, they may block areas in the uterus where an embryo could implant).

- Pain with sex (because the uterus is mobile during sex and the fibroid can press on nerves and other tissues, causing pain).
- Urinary issues (fibroids can change the shape of the uterus so that it presses on the bladder).

Adenomyosis: When tissue of the lining of the uterus grows into the uterine wall, it can cause cramping and generalized pelvic pain. It is more common in women with a history of endometriosis, and also more common in people over forty or who have had a previous procedure to their uterus, such as a D&C, an endometrial biopsy, or giving birth—it's almost like scar tissue in a way. I typically see adenomyosis in women who are in later perimenopause, because it generally takes time to form. One in three women with adenomyosis don't know they have it. Adenomyosis can sometimes be treated with medications such as birth control that stops ovulation or with a hysterectomy (the surgical removal of the uterus).

Endometriosis: This is a condition where tissue that is structurally similar to the lining of the uterus grows somewhere other than the inner uterine wall, such as upon the ovaries, fallopian tubes, or the pelvic wall. This tissue responds to hormonal fluctuations just like the lining of your uterus does, and can grow, shed, and cramp. Endometriosis usually causes pain before and during periods and contributes to heavy bleeding. It is also a risk factor for adenomyosis. It is treated with medications such as birth control that stop ovulation, or gonadotropin-releasing hormone (GnRH) agonists, such as Lupron, that work to stop the brain from producing the hormones that signal the ovaries to ovulate. Another treatment is a surgical procedure that breaks apart some of the endometrial tissue (often done with a laparoscopy) or a hysterectomy.

Uterine cancer: Uterine cancer is most commonly diagnosed in post-menopausal women in their late fifties and into their sixties. It is rarely diagnosed during perimenopause. The first sign of uterine cancer is often *post*menopausal bleeding (having a period when it has been more than one year since any bleeding). Risk factors include obesity, hypertension, diabetes, metabolic syndrome, a history of PCOS (polycystic ovary syndrome), and family history.

MEDICATIONS THAT CAN CAUSE HEAVY BLEEDING

Aspirin: Sometimes prescribed as a mild form of blood thinner for patients at risk of heart disease, aspirin can contribute to menstrual bleeding. If the risk of bleeding outweighs the benefit of the anticoagulation, then your clinician may consider stopping it.

Blood thinners: If it is medically necessary for you to be on blood thinners, such as Coumadin or Eliquis, you and your clinician may want to consider the other medications and options offered in this chapter, as blood thinners make it more difficult for your blood to form clots, which can increase bleeding—the opposite effect of what we're after.

Nonhormonal IUDs: Paragard is the one IUD that can increase bleeding. If you currently have this type of IUD and are experiencing heavy bleeding, you could consider switching to a progesterone-releasing IUD that actually stops or slows bleeding, or add one of the medications we'll discuss later to help slow or stop bleeding.

Tamoxifen: If you're taking tamoxifen for breast cancer and you are experiencing worsening bleeding, tell your doctor, as tamoxifen can slightly increase the risk of uterine cancer.

Other Possible Contributing Factors

Beyond hormones and anatomical issues like fibroids and polyps, there are a few other possible causes of heavy bleeding to consider:

- **Anovulation,** when your particular hormone fluctuations don't result in the release of an egg each month, often results in irregular menstruation. In this instance, the lining of the uterus continues to thicken until your body decides to shed it all at once. That can mean too little bleeding, or too much, and is typically outside of a predictable cycle.
- **An IUD that's been left in too long.**
- **A miscarriage.**
- **Certain bacterial infections and sexually transmitted diseases,** including trichomoniasis, chlamydia, and gonorrhea.
- **Bleeding disorders** where the blood doesn't clot very well, such as von Willebrand disease, hemophilia, and some platelet disorders.
- **Low thyroid function,** which can cause the uterine lining to grow abnormally thick, progesterone production to lessen, estrogen levels to increase, anovulation to occur, and diminish the ability to form clots to reduce the bleeding.
- **Polycystic ovary syndrome (PCOS):** Can lead to anovulatory bleeding when the message from the brain to the ovaries to release the egg doesn't work very well due to endocrine disruption.

Treatments That Can Help (in the Order I Typically Recommend Them)

If you're having a lot of bleeding, schedule an appointment with your clinician. If you were my patient, I would start by assessing your symptoms objectively, which means I'd like you to track your symptoms for a few cycles to record how many days you are bleeding, how often you are changing pads or tampons, and how it is affecting your quality of life. You can start this while you are waiting for your appointment date to arrive.

I'd also order lab work. In addition to a complete blood count (CBC) to look for anemia, I would also want to measure your levels of thyroid-stimulating hormone (TSH); free T3 and T4 (to look for subclinical hypo- or hyperthyroidism); ferritin and total iron-binding capacity (TIBC); estrogen, progesterone, and follicle-stimulating hormone (FSH, with the caveat that these levels aren't terribly helpful as they capture just a snapshot in time; still, it's good to have a record). I'd also do a pregnancy test, because a miscarriage can cause heavy bleeding, and test for bacterial infections and sexually transmitted diseases, such as trichomoniasis, gonorrhea, and chlamydia—which could be a contributing factor, just to rule out as many causes as possible.

From there, I'd suggest a pelvic exam to check for a visible cervical polyp. And I'd send you for imaging—probably an ultrasound, but maybe a CT scan or an MRI if there's a significant or concerning issue from your ultrasound.

Once we had covered these bases, you and I would discuss your possible treatment options and work together to decide what path to take from here. Unless you are going straight into the hands of a surgeon, let's discuss the medical treatment options that can help with heavy bleeding.

Progesterone-Releasing IUD (Such as the Mirena, Skyla, and Liletta)

I must confess: I am a big fan of the progesterone-releasing IUD, both for my patients and for myself. (I have had a total of three inserted, each after the birth of one of my children.) Before I tell you the specifics of the IUD, let me tell you a story about a patient of mine who is very representative of many of the perimenopausal women I see in my practice.

Kelsey is a forty-seven-year-old mother with two teenage daughters. Like a lot of women her age, Kelsey is going through perimenopause as the same time as her daughters are going through puberty—that's a lot of hormonal volatility under one roof! Her older daughter was also experiencing heavy bleeding, and her daughter's doctor had recommended going on a progesterone-only birth control pill to make her flow more manageable. When Kelsey jokingly said, "Oh, that sounds like something I could use!" the doctor told her this was a viable option for her, too. But Kelsey felt that going on the birth control pill in her mid-forties felt counterintuitive. (I get that, I really do, although since you are still able to get pregnant in perimenopause, and since birth control pills often help manage some of the symptoms of perimenopause, they can be very helpful.)

Kelsey was becoming anemic due to her heavy bleeding. In addition, she was experiencing brain fog, hair loss, and fatigue. I talked to her about the progesterone-releasing IUD, which would slow the bleeding, help bring her anemia under control, provide birth control, and hopefully help her feel more energized. On top of that, it was something that we could insert quickly, with little to no downtime on her end, and that she wouldn't have to think about again for another five years (unless she decided she wanted to have it removed before then for any reason, such as discomfort or wanting to have another child).

Kelsey was a little hesitant. She'd never had an IUD before. She was worried that it was going to hurt, but after reviewing the benefits, the convenience, and the cost (it is typically covered by insurance), she decided to go for it. While an IUD insertion is often not painful, due to her concerns, we opted to numb her cervix for the procedure. She felt crampy for a minute or two, and then nothing at all. Once the IUD was inserted, Kelsey had two light periods and then no bleeding after that. Her energy levels rebounded. And she could remove a major source of unpleasantness from her life. (We later decided to add a low-dose estradiol patch to address her brain fog and her hair loss, and I'm happy to report that those symptoms resolved, too—but we'll cover those more specifically in other chapters.)

A progesterone-releasing IUD works in two ways. Mechanically, the small T-shaped device takes up space in the uterus, making it more difficult for a fertilized egg to implant. Hormonally, the progesterone (or technically, levonorgestrel—a synthetic form of progesterone) works locally to thin the uterine lining. (See the sidebar "The Two Main Kinds of Hormone Therapy: Systemic vs. Local" for more information on what I mean by working locally.) Basically, an IUD works by making your uterus inhospitable to a fertilized egg.

Its list of benefits is robust: In addition to slowing or even stopping bleeding, it has been shown to decrease the risk of endometrial and ovarian cancer when used for at least four years.[3] It is also highly effective as birth control, and the progesterone it releases can serve as the progesterone arm of your hormone therapy (as anyone with a uterus who takes supplemental estrogen also needs to take progesterone to protect the uterus from cancer risk). On top of that, an IUD is not *quite* set it and forget it, but it's close—you can leave it in for at least five years, and once placed you should not even be able to tell it's there. (If you can feel it, it probably means that part of it is in the cervix and it needs to be removed and reinserted, as it's not in the right place.)

There is only one IUD that doesn't release progesterone—the Paragard, which contains copper wires wrapped around the plastic core of the device. It can actually increase bleeding and cramping, especially in the first three to six months. Not generally what we're after in perimenopause, so, for this use, it should be avoided.

There are a few myths about progesterone-releasing IUDs.

Myth 1: It's painful to insert. Reference the sidebar "Is Getting an IUD Painful?"

Myth 2: It increases the risk of ectopic pregnancy. In fact, IUDs decrease this risk because they decrease the risk of pregnancy in general.

Myth 3: It increases the risk of pelvic inflammatory disease (PID). This has been fully debunked, in particular by a study that followed nearly sixty thousand women for ninety days after receiving an IUD, showing a risk of developing PID of less than 1 percent.[4]

Myth 4: It could easily fall out. This risk is extremely low and rises only if you get the IUD placed right after giving birth or having a pregnancy termination. However, I had mine placed right after my daughter was born and it stayed right where it was supposed to be!

Myth 5: It's for younger women, or just for birth control. It absolutely can be used as part of your HT regimen even once you are menopausal, although it is currently not FDA-approved for that reason, so it is used off-label. It's also great for anyone who has an intolerance to progesterone, which about one-third of patients do. (I'll talk more about this in chapter 5, but the short version is, some women feel either super tired, bloated, or moody when taking oral progesterone.)

IS GETTING AN IUD PAINFUL?

As someone who both inserts IUDs as a clinician and has had IUDs inserted, I can tell you from experience that many women do not experience pain or discomfort during the insertion process or after, but there are always exceptions. Your health history may play a role in your experience, as research suggests that women who have had one or more vaginal births experience less pain than women who haven't.[5]

While the uterus doesn't have a lot of nerve endings (which is a good thing, considering how much the uterus expands and contracts each menstrual cycle—not to mention during pregnancy and birth), the cervix does. Since the IUD must pass through the cervix to reach the uterus, pain is definitely a possibility, and is often due to various nerves in the two- to three-centimeter-long cervical canal.

For many years women's pain has been ignored in general, including during IUD insertions. The good news is that in 2024 the Centers for Disease Control and Prevention updated their guidelines to recommend that doctors discuss pain management options before an IUD insertion and use shared decision-making with their patients to choose a course of action. This change was largely the result of many women posting videos on social media of their painful reactions to getting an IUD. (Go, women!)

The other good news is that we know from research that an injection of lidocaine—a localized pain reliever similar to the novocaine you get at the dentist—is very effective at reducing the pain, and more effective than over-the-counter painkillers such as naproxen or ibuprofen. One downside is that the shot itself may be painful. There are also lidocaine creams, gels, and sprays.

Some doctors consider any kind of pain relief an unnecessary step because it's really quick to insert an IUD and it can take awhile for the numbing to take effect, and that numbing can be uncomfortable. But you deserve the opportunity to discuss your options for pain relief and to feel like your doctor is engaging in shared decision-making to help you choose.

Depo-Provera

Technically a form of birth control, Depo-Provera injections can also slow heavy bleeding over time. Comprised of medroxyprogesterone acetate—a synthetic form of progesterone—Depo-Provera suppresses ovulation, which then also diminishes the buildup and the shedding of the uterine lining. It works because steady progesterone blocks the surge of both luteinizing hormone (LH) and estrogen that typically happens in the first half of your cycle (known as the luteal phase), meaning the signals that cue ovulation aren't received.

You will need to get an injection four times a year—otherwise, the shot is convenient; you won't need to regularly pick up meds or remember to take a pill each day. I have to tell you, just as I tell all my patients, that some studies have shown moderate weight gain (up to ten pounds) with Depo. I hate to bring it up because this scares many women away from the possibility. The FDA has also issued a warning that Depo-Provera can cause significant bone loss—for this reason, you don't want to use it for more than a few years, but that could be just enough time to get you through the worst of your heavy bleeding and perhaps even into your menopausal transition.[6] With the Depo shot, your injection site may be sore for a day or two, but otherwise, there's no long healing period. Most people begin to see results—lessened bleeding—within two or three cycles.

THE TWO MAIN KINDS OF HORMONE THERAPY: SYSTEMIC VS. LOCAL

Not all hormonal treatments act the same within the body. Some stay put and affect only the tissues that they are applied to directly—these are called local treatments. And others get into the bloodstream and have effects throughout the body— these are systemic.

Systemic: Birth control patch; birth control ring (NuvaRing); birth control pills; Prometrium (bioidentical FDA-approved form of postmenopausal progesterone in oral capsules); testosterone cream or gel; Femring (a vaginal ring that delivers systemic estradiol)

Local: IUD (which contains levonorgestrel, a form of progestin); vaginal estrogen (creams, suppositories); Estring (a vaginal ring that delivers local estradiol)

Systemic Delivery	Local Delivery
The hormone is distributed throughout the entire body	The hormone is directly applied at the target zone

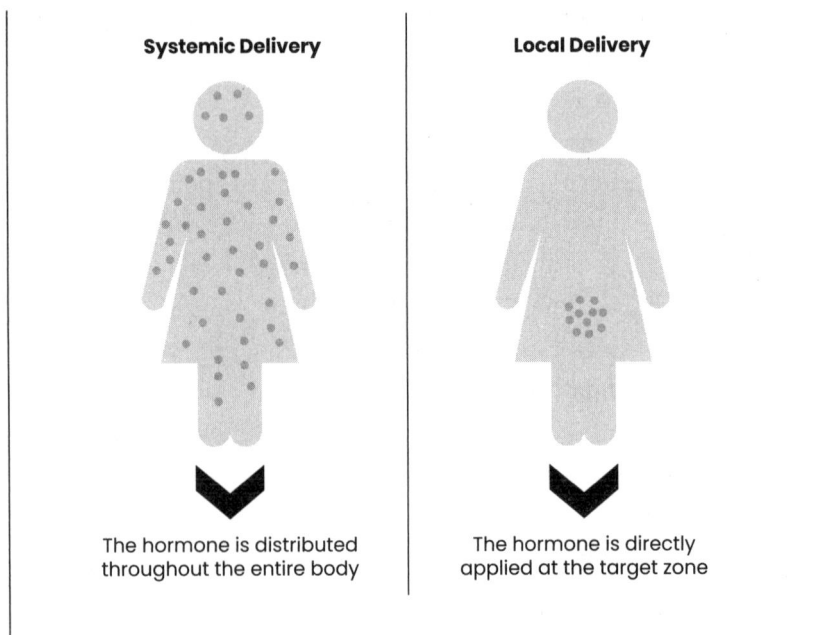

Progesterone-Only Oral Birth Control (Sometimes Called the "Mini Pill")

This progesterone-only form of birth control pill—technically, norethindrone, a synthetic progestin—thins the cervical mucus and the uterine lining, both of which make it very unlikely that a sperm will fertilize an egg, or that a fertilized egg will implant in the uterus. It may also stop ovulation—although about half of people using the mini pill do still ovulate—and with no egg released, the uterus does not get the cue to build up its lining.[7] And, of course, it's also birth control, although, instead of birth control pills, I like to call them "perimenopause pills," especially when heavy bleeding is your primary symptom, as it was for Daria.

Daria was forty-four, and her monthly bleeding was terrible. So were her mood swings. Her libido was barely a blip. Part of the reason her bleeding was so heavy was that she had several fibroids, which meant she wasn't a candidate for an IUD. Daria also wanted to avoid surgery if possible. Even though her partner had a vasectomy and she didn't technically need birth control, through shared decision-making Daria opted to try the mini pills. Within two cycles, she was down to two days of manageable bleeding and one day of spotting per month. Once she stabilized, we added topical testosterone, which helped her libido rise—and she noticed her mood stabilized, too. You can start the pills at any point during your cycle, and it should take four to eight weeks to reach peak effectiveness.

Combined Oral Contraceptives, Taken Continuously

"Combined" here means that the birth control pills contain both a synthetic progesterone (typically in the form of norethindrone or drospirenone) and estrogen (in the form of ethinyl estradiol), meaning they can not only stop ovulation but also potentially reduce symptoms of lowering estrogen (such as hot flashes, night sweats, and vaginal dryness). Combined oral contraceptives have been found to be protective of bone health when taken in the perimenopause years (the opposite is typically true for teenage girls).[8] Plus, obviously, they offer contraception and pregnancy is still a possibility in perimenopause.

Many birth control pills include seven days of placebo pills to mimic a monthly cycle and give your uterus a chance to expel any minimal lining it may have built up. When you skip the placebo pills and take the pills continuously, you typically forgo all bleeding, although you may have some light spotting or breakthrough bleeding. Combined contraceptives may take a few monthly cycles to adjust, reaching full effectiveness in four to eight weeks.

SIDE EFFECTS AND CONTRAINDICATIONS TO BIRTH CONTROL PILLS

Birth control pills can be quite effective in managing the symptoms of perimenopause—there's a reason why I think of them as "perimenopause pills." But, like any prescription medication, they aren't a silver bullet. Here is a tour of their side effects and the reasons why they may not be a suitable choice for you.[9]

Potential side effects of both types of birth control pills—progesterone-only and combined:

- Breast tenderness.
- Lower testosterone levels, which is good for alleviating acne, but can also lead to a lowering of libido as well as vaginal dryness, because the vagina is rich in androgen receptors as well as estrogen receptors.
- Mood changes (not proven, but my patients report it).
- Nausea.
- Slightly increased risk of blood clots. The average baseline risk of a woman developing a blood clot is 3 in 10,000 women. For women on oral birth control, the average risk is 9 in 10,000. To put these risks in perspective, if you're pregnant, the average risk is 15 in 10,000.[10]
- Spotting between periods and may cause irregular bleeding—so sometimes it's not the right treatment for heavy bleeding.
- Water retention.
- Weight gain—although not scientifically proven, there is some anecdotal evidence that birth control pills cause weight gain, but most specifically the Depo-Provera injection has been shown to cause up to ten pounds of weight gain in some women.

Contraindications for progesterone-only birth control pills:

- Breast cancer.
- Certain anti-seizure medications.
- Liver disease.
- Personal history of bariatric surgery.
- Pregnancy.
- Undiagnosed abnormal uterine bleeding.

Contraindications for combined oral contraceptives:

- Heavy smoking if you are over age thirty-five.
- Migraines with aura.
- Personal history of estrogen-sensitive cancer, including breast and endometrial.
- Personal history of deep vein thrombosis.
- Personal history of heart disease, including atrial fibrillation, stroke, subacute bacterial endocarditis.
- Significant liver disease.
- Uncontrolled high blood pressure.
- Uncontrolled diabetes.

Endometrial Ablation

This procedure involves cauterizing the lining of the uterus, generally using heat, scarring the uterine lining so it grows back less thickly, and therefore there is less of it to shed.

An ablation is less invasive than a hysterectomy, but it does have its downsides. It may not work completely, and it can make it harder to get a good sample to assess uterine pathology if you have a need to do so later. Ablation can also greatly impede your chance of getting pregnant or carrying that pregnancy to term if you do decide later that you want to conceive. If you want to keep the door to pregnancy propped open, this is not the treatment for you.

Like hysterectomies, ablations are less popular than they once were due to the effectiveness and relative ease of IUDs to control heavy bleeding. You'll need one to two days to heal, with peak effectiveness building over a few months.

Uterine Artery Embolization (UAE)

This outpatient procedure is performed by an interventional radiologist, who uses a catheter to place small particles inside the blood vessels that lead to the uterus, blocking blood flow. A UAE can be used as a treatment for fibroids—when the fibroids are denied a blood supply, they shrink—or can be used to treat heavy bleeding in general. With these arteries cut off, the lining of the uterus doesn't get the blood it would need to grow, and, therefore, you don't develop a lining that then needs to be shed. Because this procedure is more involved, you may feel better in a few days but should give yourself one to two weeks to fully heal. You'll see either a significant decline in or a cessation of bleeding in two to three months.

Hysterectomy

A hysterectomy is the removal of the uterus, a procedure that can be done a few different ways—laproscopically, vaginally, or through an abdominal opening—and can remove different amounts of tissue—the uterus, the uterus and cervix combined, or the uterus, cervix, and supporting structures around the uterus. It is important to note that a hysterectomy does not include the removal of the fallopian tubes or ovaries. If that is included in your hysterectomy, it is called a hysterectomy with bilateral salpingo-oophorectomy. While we're on the topic, there is no need to remove the ovaries for the sole reason of heavy bleeding; there should be another solid reason to do so as removing the ovaries will put you into surgical menopause (immediately after surgery you will experience menopause).

According to a 2024 CDC report (based on 2021 numbers), 22.1 percent of American women between the ages of forty-five and sixty-five have had a hysterectomy.[11] A hysterectomy was long considered the go-to solution for a range of issues, including fibroids, heavy bleeding, uterine cancer treatment as well as uterine and cervical cancer prevention, and endometriosis. Now, there are many alternative treatment options available for all of these conditions. Although hysterectomy rates have been declining as a result, it is still the second-most-common surgery in women, after cesarean sections. About six hundred thousand hysterectomies are performed on women every year.

Because a hysterectomy is irreversible and can mean major surgery, with weeks of downtime and a small but still significant risk of complications, I usually suggest patients try a reversible medical intervention first. That said, it really depends on your symptoms, quality of life, health history, and circumstances. I've seen women begging to have their uterus removed so they can be done with the bleeding once and for all, and their doctor brushing them off. I've also talked to many women who aren't interested though their surgeons are advocating for it. Every woman deserves a shot at medical management and to be given the gift of shared decision-making. The IUD in particular has proven to be so effective, in addition to being reversible, with very little if any downtime, and low in cost—it is definitely worthy of at least your serious consideration before you opt for a hysterectomy if your primary issue is heavy bleeding.

Each method has different recovery times, but a general recommendation is that women take off work for six weeks after a hysterectomy, although you will need to make sure you're moving regularly during the healing process to prevent blood clots. It will be several weeks before bleeding fully stops.

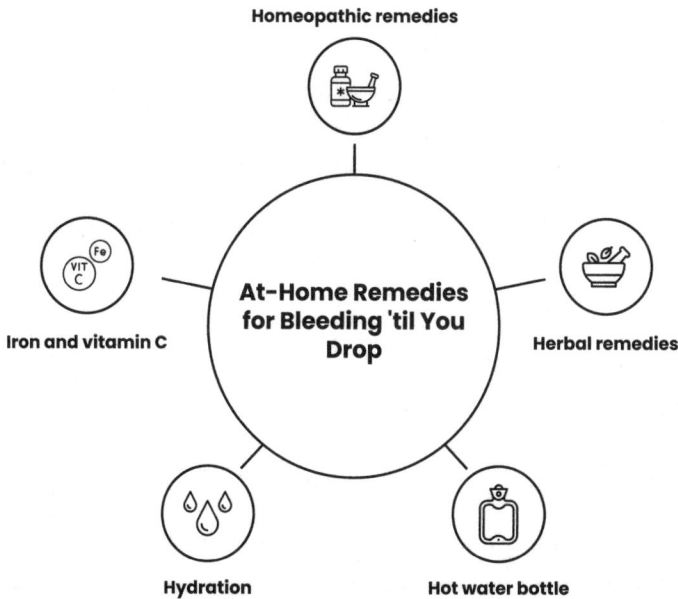

Homeopathic remedies

Iron and vitamin C

At-Home Remedies for Bleeding 'til You Drop

Herbal remedies

Hydration

Hot water bottle

What You Can Do on Your Own

This is one symptom set that typically requires some level of medical intervention to fully resolve, yet there are many things you can do to support yourself through intense periods of bleeding.

Herbal Remedies

There are herbs that have a track record and some data to support their effectiveness in reducing heavy menstrual bleeding, including:

- **Ginger.** Ginger has been hailed for centuries for its anti-inflammatory effects and digestive benefits. It seems to also be helpful at reducing heavy bleeding. One randomized, double-blind, placebo-controlled study found that women with heavy bleeding who took 250 mg of dried ginger in capsule form three times a day, starting on the day before the beginning of their period through the third day of bleeding, saw a 46 percent decrease in bleeding, compared to only a 2 percent decrease in the placebo group.[12]
- **Raspberry leaf tea.** A known uterine tonic—often suggested for pregnant women because it strengthens the muscles of the uterine wall—raspberry leaf tea is also high in iron, so it can help replenish your iron stores as it supports your uterus. Steep the leaves to make a tea and drink a cup or two a day the week before and during your period.
- **Yarrow** (*Achillea millefolium*). Yarrow has been used traditionally to treat bleeding and speed wound healing because of its astringent (drying) properties. It's also antispasmodic and anti-inflammatory, which means it should help reduce cramping, too. Look for it in tincture form at your local health food store, and take a half-dropperful every three hours while on your period.

Homeopathic Remedies

Homeopathy is a traditional form of medicine where very small doses of a plant-based remedy are administered to send a message to the body.

It is based on the principle of "like cures like," meaning each remedy actually causes the symptoms it's seeking to alleviate, but such a small dose is given that the body's healing response is elicited to that symptom without experiencing the full-blown reaction. I think of it like an herbal vaccine. Homeopathic remedies are available in most drugstores. The three homeopathic remedies that are recommended to treat heavy perimenopausal bleeding are belladonna (especially if you experience heat and a sensation of fullness in the pelvis with your bleeding); black cohosh (*Cimicifuga racemosa*), which is recommended for women with irregular, painful periods and is also said to help with moodiness and depressive symptoms that stem from hormonal swings; and sabina (particularly if you are passing a lot of dark clots and feeling lower back pain, or your bleeding gets worse when you move).

Other Options
There are other things you can do to support yourself through this time as you partner with a doctor to find the treatment that's appropriate to you.

- **Support your iron levels** by taking iron supplements and prioritizing iron-rich and vitamin C–rich foods since vitamin C promotes iron absorption. Consult with your doctor before you take iron pills, because your hemoglobin levels can be tested to see if you do need extra iron and if so, to guide your dosage. Iron-rich foods include: beans, beef, beets, clams, lamb, lentils, liver, mussels, pumpkin seeds, stewed tomatoes, spinach, Swiss chard, turkey, and oysters. Great sources of vitamin C include: broccoli, brussels sprouts, cantaloupe, guava, kale, kiwi, lemons, oranges, papaya, parsley, strawberries, and yellow bell peppers.
- **Prioritize hydration** by drinking plenty of water and eating water-rich foods like fruits and vegetables, as this will help you keep your blood volume up (which can dip when you are bleeding heavily). Top high-water-content foods include: apples, bell

peppers, cantaloupe, cauliflower, celery, cucumber, lettuce, oranges, peaches, strawberries, tomatoes, watermelon, and zucchini.

- **Soothe cramps** by applying a hot water bottle or heating pad to your abdomen, which will help relax the uterine muscles. Plus, it just feels nice.

Once you've addressed your heavy bleeding, it's time to move on to your next most bothersome symptom set.

CHAPTER 5

Lying Awake and Worrying

Jennifer, a forty-six-year-old single mother of two and a physical therapist, was exhausted at the end of the day. Yet whenever she got into bed, she had trouble falling asleep because she couldn't stop thinking about her to-do list, her bills, and her teenage daughter, who was dating someone she felt was a bad influence. She'd never really thought of herself as an anxious person before, but now it was like her brain couldn't shut off. Although Jennifer had always been a good sleeper, she started dreading going to bed because of the new onset of nighttime worrying, tossing, and turning. To make matters worse, her lost sleep was making her irritable and fuzzy-headed. Jennifer felt like she wasn't being a great parent, and she knew her performance at work was falling off, which only added to her anxiety.

Aniyah has always worked in a high-stress environment—she currently makes her living jumping out of planes as a professional skydiver, of all things!—and up until recently had managed just fine. But once she turned forty-four, her heart began racing and fluttering, which sent her anxiety spiraling. She started waking up in the middle of the night and tossing and turning, imagining various worst-case scenarios that got her so worked up she rarely fell back to sleep. Aniyah saw a psychiatrist to change her antidepressant (it didn't help); made an appointment with a cardiologist (who said her heart function was normal); and gave up caffeine because she thought maybe it was playing a role in making her feel so jittery (which only made her feel more tired).

Both of these women were struggling with the "lying awake and worrying" symptom set, even though they each had slightly different presentations. Later in this chapter I'll share the treatments and approaches they each used to get back on board the good-sleep train. But before we dive into remedies, let's take a closer look at why these symptoms are so problematic and why they tend to be so common in women at midlife.

LYING AWAKE AND WORRYING AT A GLANCE

Symptoms:

- Poor sleep, whether that's difficulty falling asleep, staying asleep, or both
- An uptick in anxious thoughts (often before bed, but can strike at any time)
- Periodically feeling like your heart is racing or skipping a beat
- Fatigue
- Brain fog
- Irritability

Causative factors:

- Low progesterone, and the resulting decrease of gamma-aminobutyric acid (GABA), a neurotransmitter that calms neuronal excitability and inhibits nerve transmission in the central nervous system (CNS)
- Volatile estrogen levels
- Reduced alcohol tolerance
- Poor sleep hygiene

The Risks of Lying Awake and Worrying

Sleeplessness is the chicken to anxiety's egg: Can you not get to sleep because you're anxious, or are you anxious because you can't get enough restorative sleep? In perimenopause, these two related symptoms are incredibly common—70 percent of my patients report racing thoughts and trouble sleeping. It truly can be a vicious cycle that gets worse as the anxiety starts to tick up more and more the closer you get to bedtime, and then the insomnia causes brain fog, exhaustion, low mood, low energy, and frustration during the day. You can easily imagine this vicious cycle getting worse and worse over time.

On a deeper level, sleep is a fundamental pillar of health. Poor sleep can lead to significant health problems, including a decline in cognitive function and a rise in the risk of depression and metabolic syndrome—the triad of high blood pressure, high blood sugar, and high cholesterol that is associated with heart disease, the number one killer of women. If you are feeling tired and stressed all the time, it can also breed isolation, which is a health risk on its own.

Sleep is absolutely fundamental to health. This statement was confirmed by a 2023 study that evaluated the sleep of nearly 175,000 adults ages eighteen and older. The results showed that women who slept seven to eight hours per night, had difficulty falling asleep or staying asleep less than twice per week, did not take sleep medications, and woke up feeling rested at least five days per week had a life expectancy that was nearly two and a half years longer than women who didn't.[1] Yet sleep is one area of health where there is a big disparity between genders. According to a 2023 survey by the American Academy of Sleep Medicine, women are twice as likely as men to report that they rarely feel well-rested.[2] Researchers from Cambridge University also found that women tend to sleep about eleven minutes less than men each night, although they are typically in bed fifteen minutes longer.[3] This means women are spending more time lying awake, probably counting how many hours of sleep we can expect to get if we could only fall back to sleep, or worrying, or replaying the stressful situations we lived through earlier that day.

When nighttime anxiety and insomnia start during perimenopause—or perhaps they started during pregnancy and the early, sleepless years of parenthood, only to become further cemented once perimenopause arrives on the scene—they can kick off years (if not decades) of poor sleep. These detriments to good sleep slowly build up to the point that a bad night's sleep becomes the norm. Without intervention, this cycle won't get better on its own, even after you're on the other side of menopause.

To make matters more uncertain, it's hard to know where to turn. A therapist? Psychiatrist? Primary care doctor? Sleep doctor? Cardiologist? The sad truth is that without this book, you could schedule appointments with all of them and likely never get confirmation that your symptoms are hormonally related—or the help that addressing the hormone imbalances causing your symptoms can provide.

Not to be dramatic, but the poor sleep that occurs now can continue for the rest of your life if you don't take steps to course-correct. I understand that women are still statistically likely to be putting in more hours of housework than men, while also carrying a heavier mental load in regard to doing the majority of planning for the family and keeping track of what needs to be purchased and done. While these truths are maddening, they do help explain why we women often feel that we have fewer hours to devote to rest, and a harder time quieting our minds when we do get in bed. Despite all the societal and physiological reasons why you may be feeling anxious and tired, your ability to sleep is not permanently broken. It *can* get better, especially when you understand the root causes of poor sleep in perimenopause and take steps to address them, which is exactly what I'll walk you through in this chapter.

What Causes Sleeplessness and Anxiety in Perimenopause

There are two driving factors behind this symptom set: hormonal decline, and poor sleep habits. In order to turn the tide on your current sleep trajectory, you need to tend to both of these factors.

The decline in both estrogen and progesterone plays a role. In general, having trouble falling asleep is a sign of low progesterone, while difficulty staying asleep tends to be low estrogen.

Let's start with progesterone. In addition to regulating the uterine lining, progesterone is a calming hormone. It surges in the first trimester of pregnancy—in part to support the development of the placenta, and in part to keep a mother relaxed and able to rest during this vulnerable, crucial stage in pregnancy. When progesterone starts to decline in perimenopause, our sleep naturally gets a little lighter and our thoughts can get a little louder, making it more difficult to fall asleep and much easier to feel anxious.

Progesterone also increases the production of gamma-aminobutyric acid (GABA), a neurotransmitter that helps you relax, feel sleepy, and fall asleep. GABA is an inhibitory neurotransmitter, which means it slows brain activity by blocking signals in the central nervous system. It's like the brakes in your car, but slowing information in the brain and nervous system to keep you from getting overwhelmed. Progesterone is broken down into chemicals, including allopregnanolone, which also increase GABA production.

Low estrogen causes middle-of-the-night waking because estrogen helps to control the variability of your internal thermostat. It doesn't change your core body temperature, but it gives you more of a flexible range to quickly adapt to changes in ambient temp. As estrogen declines, that temperature variability window gets smaller, so that then when your body heat builds up under one too many blankets, or your partner just breathes on you, it can wake you up. Or maybe you're having full-blown hot flashes and night sweats. Either way, once you're up, your brain is on and you're worrying.

In addition, the estrogen volatility that is a hallmark of perimenopause is a well-established cause of heart palpitations. Couple an uncomfortable fluttering in your chest with anxiety, and it's a perfect storm for a full-blown panic attack. For many of my patients, their first panic attack has landed them in the ER because they were (rightfully) worried they were having a heart attack.

On the sleep-habit side, many of us in our late thirties and forties typically don't have great sleep habits because up until our hormones started changing, we've been able to easily fall asleep and stay asleep. Now, in midlife, there's a lot to worry about. Plus, some of the things we used to do without thinking twice—having a couple of glasses of wine with dinner chief among them—are now contributing to our wakefulness. Alcohol is metabolized in the liver, as are our hormones. If your liver is busy—which it can be after a decade or two of having to process a nightly glass of alcohol—it gets less effective at breaking down estrogens, meaning you have even less of it on hand working in the body. And low estrogen is an invitation for hot flashes and night sweats, which explains why alcohol can be a hot flash trigger.

Many of the things we use to try to help us sleep better actually make the problem worse. Perhaps you haven't been aware of the connection between alcohol and wakefulness, and you've been trying to help yourself sleep by self-medicating with wine. Or maybe you're trying to ensure you'll be knocked out enough to sleep by taking Tylenol PM, melatonin, cannabis, Benadryl, or sleep meds, which generally leave you feeling drowsy and hungover the next morning, and more importantly, leave you even further away from learning how to put yourself to sleep. Plus, they don't address the fundamental root of the problem, which is, in part, our declining hormones.

A COMMON, YET UNDERDISCUSSED, MIDLIFE PHENOMENON: HEALTH-CARE-RELATED ANXIETY

Perimenopause, with its rotating cast of characters of symptoms that can seem as if they have come out of nowhere, is a common time for a specific kind of anxiety to take root: a pressing and persistent worry about your health. Although many women have various health issues to manage throughout their lives, perimenopause is often the first time, outside of obstetrics, that women start utilizing the health-care system. They often just haven't had a reason to see a doctor with any regularity. If this is familiar to you, you can feel like you are going from zero to one hundred in terms of worrying about your health and wellness.

Then the symptoms start—whether it's more frequent UTIs, headaches, or migraines; or the first time you're experiencing back pain or fatigue that you don't seem to back bounce from. Maybe you're having difficulty remembering things and noticing that your heart sometimes races. It's often the first time you realize that you've been taking your general wellness for granted. And it's so easy to get on the internet and go down a rabbit hole, self-diagnosing yourself with every scary-sounding condition imaginable. All of this may also coincide with a time of life when you may be losing someone you love, you're really involved at work, you have family demands to deal with, and you're not sleeping that well . . . it's the perfect-storm opportunity for health-related anxiety to bloom.

Perhaps one month you have breast tenderness and you can't stop thinking about it or looking up all the reasons you might have it. You read something that lists breast tenderness as a symptom of breast cancer and then you're researching stats and treatments. The next month you leave your purse behind in three different places and can't remember a friend's name when you run into her, and then you're looking up signs of early-onset Alzheimer's. We all check in with Dr. Google every once in a while (and likely see something that scares us), but if you're going on a wild ride of fear and research repeatedly, it might be time to talk to a mental health provider about how to break the cycle. I know the worry may feel protective, but it is also a form of stress, which is not going to help your symptoms get better. Beyond that, time you spend continually researching ways you could be dying is time you're *not living*. Reclaim that time and energy and put it toward activities that will make you feel better, whether that's getting some movement, talking with a friend, or doing something that brings you joy.

If this is something you've been experiencing, remember the health-care adage that "common things happen commonly." Perimenopause is not only common, it's universal. Almost everyone born with ovaries will go through perimenopause, and chances are very good that changing hormones are contributing to your symptoms, no matter how unrelated they may seem. This is yet another reason to start journaling and tracking your symptoms so you can identify patterns and determine if there's a specific area, such as diet, sleep, mental health, or exercise, where you could make improvements. Stay out of the online rabbit hole so you can stop imagining various worst-case scenarios. A cognitive behavioral therapy (CBT) technique I find helpful is to schedule my worry time, giving myself twenty minutes to either journal what I'm worried about, talk it out with a friend or my husband or my therapist, or do some online research. That means you don't have to be thinking about what's worrying you all the time, and when you do think about it, you're setting some limits for yourself. Also, start the search for a hormone-savvy clinician if you don't already have one.

Treatments That Can Help (in the Order I Typically Recommend Them)

Progesterone

Because so many of the symptoms in this set—especially difficulty falling asleep and feeling anxious—are driven by declining levels of progesterone, my first choice is usually to add progesterone back in the form of the bioidentical, FDA-approved Prometrium. I generally recommend starting with a dose of 100 mg taken at bedtime. (Prometrium is mixed with peanut oil, so if you have a peanut allergy, your doctor may need to have a special blend made for you by a compounding pharmacy.) Sometimes 100 mg isn't sufficient for sleep, so you may try increasing that to 200 mg. The maximum dose I prescribe is 400 mg. You can either take Prometrium every night, or take it only on the twelve days in the second half of your cycle, when progesterone is now declining. How often you take it in perimenopause should be dictated by your symptoms. If you have trouble sleeping only the five nights before your period, you could take it for just half the month. If you need help sleeping most nights, you could take it continuously. Once you are in menopause, work closely with your clinician to determine how often you should take progesterone in order to protect against uterine cancer.

Based on her symptoms, Jennifer and I decided to prioritize improving her sleep and reducing her anxiety. She left my office with a prescription for oral progesterone, and after just a few nights she was already sleeping better and feeling less anxious. She also resolved to get in bed right around the same time each night, to start wearing a sleep mask to block out light, and to add in a few minutes of either stretching or journaling to her wind-down routine. By her follow-up appointment three months later, she reported feeling much better rested and more productive at her job.

One note of caution: As I covered in chapter 2, over-the-counter progesterone creams don't provide a sufficient dosage to physiologically replace progesterone because progesterone is a big molecule, which means it's not easily absorbed through the skin. They may give a placebo effect, but they're not an efficient form of hormone therapy. If you're also taking estradiol, OTC progesterone creams won't provide enough protection for the uterus.

IF PROGESTERONE DOESN'T AGREE WITH YOU

As helpful as progesterone can be for lowering anxiety and promoting more restful sleep, some women don't tolerate it well. In my clinical practice, approximately one-third of women find that progesterone causes side effects, with some patients complaining of excessive drowsiness, while others may experience bloating.

If lying awake and worrying is your primary symptom set, you could try a different formulation or delivery method for your progesterone. For example, if oral progesterone makes you feel bloated, you could try using either an intravaginal or transdermal in the form of an FDA-approved combined estrogen-progesterone patch. Progesterone via these delivery systems would bypass the digestive system and perhaps relieve you from the digestive side effects, too. Or you could try a synthetic progesterone, such as Aygestin (or norethindrone), as a different formulation may give you a different experience. But since the first and foremost aim of any kind of hormone therapy is to resolve symptoms, if a treatment is creating symptoms of its own, it's time to try something else, such as cognitive behavioral therapy for insomnia (we'll discuss this shortly), or some of the lifestyle interventions that have been shown to improve sleep in perimenopause that I outline starting on page 106.

Estradiol

If your sleep issues are more of the can't *stay* asleep variety—meaning, you drift off just fine but find yourself waking up in the middle of the night and struggle to get back to sleep—adding supplemental estrogen may help. That's because a hallmark symptom of declining estrogen is night sweats, which are notorious for waking women up. For some women, this means waking up drenched in sweat. But you don't need a full-blown hot flash attack to wake you up. Body temperature is a big piece of sleep (room temperature should be around sixty-five degrees or less for optimal sleeping conditions), and since estrogen helps the brain to regulate an overall lower body temperature, when it starts declining you can run hot. A patient of mine describes it as feeling like a baked potato that someone left in the oven a little too long. And it's hard to sleep when you're overheated.

It'll be important to work with a clinician to determine dosing as well as timing—maybe, in perimenopause, you experience difficulty sleeping the seven to ten days before your period starts. In that case, you may need to supplement with estradiol during only those days. This may be the only medical treatment you need to start sleeping better, although everyone can benefit from getting their sleep hygiene dialed in.

Something else to keep in mind is that when you are postmenopausal, taking estradiol, and still have a uterus, you also need to take progesterone to protect yourself from uterine cancer. Since you are still perimenopausal (i.e., it has not been at least a year since your last period), you are likely still making some progesterone, so it is okay to take estradiol alone without countering it with progesterone until the time between periods lengthens to two or three months. By the time you go one year without a period, you definitely need to update your HT plan to add a stable dose of progesterone to your regimen to reduce any risk of uterine cancer.

Aniyah, who had been feeling extremely anxious, spending most of the middle of the night awake, and experiencing heart palpitations, finally showed up at my office after a friend suggested that maybe hormones were to blame. Because she was waking up in the middle of the night more frequently (which tends to be the result of declining estrogen) and her heart was racing (which can also be triggered by volatile levels of estrogen), we started her on an estradiol patch. It helped her heartbeat stabilize, which removed a big source of anxiety. She also adjusted her sleep routine a bit. On those nights when she woke up, instead of tossing and turning in bed she'd go lie on her couch, wrap herself in a cozy blanket and listen to a sleep podcast (a podcast designed to be just boring enough to help you get drowsy and just interesting enough to hold your attention so your thoughts don't spiral). After a little while she'd feel sleepy again—only then would she get back into bed (a tactic you'll learn more about in the "build up your sleep hunger" bullet later in this chapter). Aniyah also realized her nightly post-dinner glass of wine was contributing to her night wakings, so she swapped it out for a cup of rooibos chai (a caffeine-free herbal tea). This combination of treatment and lifestyle changes helped her settle into a new pattern of getting a solid seven to eight hours of sleep a night.

Cognitive Behavioral Therapy for Insomnia (CBT-I)

Cognitive behavioral therapy (CBT) is a form of psychological treatment that helps to objectively identify thoughts and behaviors that may be causing issues and then modify them to create new patterns of behavior or habits that are more helpful. If you've been to or are currently in therapy, you may already be familiar. There is a form of CBT specifically designed to help with sleeplessness called CBT-I, the "I" standing for insomnia. On the cognitive side, CBT-I helps you to find and then change beliefs, negative thoughts, and worries that prevent you from sleeping. On the behavioral side, CBT-I guides you through adopting good sleep habits and practicing relaxation techniques. CBT has also been found to be effective in managing hot flashes by coaching you to breathe slowly from your belly (known as paced breathing) while allowing the rising heat to wash over you, so if night sweats are part of your insomnia equation, CBT can help with them, too.

CBT-I has great data to support its effectiveness. Research has found that as many as 80 percent of people with insomnia enjoy benefits including more sleep time overall, taking less time to fall asleep, and waking up fewer times during the night. Most importantly, these benefits are long-lasting.[4] For the full CBT-I experience, search the websites of the Society of Behavioral Sleep Medicine or the American Board of Sleep Medicine. Treatment generally lasts from six to eight sessions. There are also many apps that will lead you through CBT-I exercises, including CBT-i Coach, Stellar Sleep, Sleep Reset, and Sleepio, some of which are free.

If you want to try out a CBT-I technique as early as tonight, here are some of the cognitive behavioral therapy–based strategies I practice on nights when I'm having trouble sleeping:

- I remind myself that I have yet to solve a major problem at 2:30 a.m., and that reminder helps me set the worries aside.

- I tell myself I'll have a twenty-minute worry period in the morning, when I'll write down all the things that are troubling me. Even though I may not actually sit down and do it once I'm awake, it helps me let those worries go, at least for a little while.
- I will play a little game with myself, such as taking a mental tour through all the places I've lived, remembering the details of past vacations, or figuring out where I would choose to go if I were going to eat out for the next three nights. You could also mentally list all the things you're grateful for, or what went well that day, or what you're looking forward to tomorrow.

Certain Antidepressant or Antianxiety Medications

As a physician who specializes in treating perimenopausal and menopausal symptoms, I can't help but suspect that declining hormones are a root cause of symptoms that either present or worsen for women in their perimenopausal years, and I do typically recommend hormonal solutions first. But let's not forget that sleeplessness and worry can be symptoms of generalized anxiety disorder (GAD) or depression, which means that medications in the selective serotonin reuptake inhibitor (SSRI) and serotonin-norepinephrine reuptake inhibitor (SNRI) classes may be helpful.

There has been a history of doctors who want to help women but haven't been adequately trained about perimenopause and thus suggest antidepressants or antianxiety meds first when women ask for help with their fatigue, worry, or sleeplessness. I hear from so many women that it can feel like a dismissal—like you're earnestly seeking help for a legitimate concern and your doctor is suggesting your symptoms are all in your head. Although there has never been a trial that compares the effectiveness of hormone therapy vs. mood medications in relieving perimenopausal symptoms—and I very much look forward to the day that we have this kind of data—I'm inclined to try hormone therapy first to see if your sleeplessness and worrying get better. If they do, it strongly suggests that the underlying cause was hormones, and not a mood disorder.

That being said, if you have tried hormone therapy and that didn't completely work to resolve your sleep issues, it may be time to consider an alternative diagnosis such as depression or anxiety and therefore a different treatment. Also, many women have found SSRIs or SNRIs to be helpful for sleep and anxiety, and if that approach makes more sense for you than hormone therapy for whatever reason, by all means, take that help. This class of medications may very well help stop the nighttime ruminating thoughts—trying to solve everyone's problems in your family, strategizing how to position your side of an argument, remembering all the people you need to call. You're still going to need to bump up your sleep hygiene!

At-Home Remedies for Lying Awake and Worrying

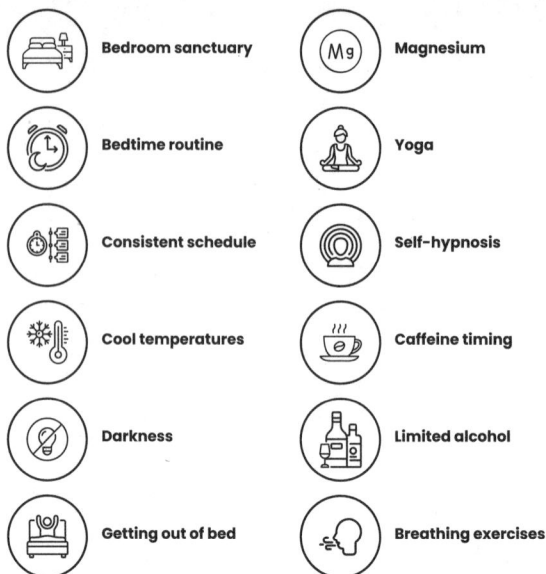

Bedroom sanctuary   Magnesium

Bedtime routine   Yoga

Consistent schedule   Self-hypnosis

Cool temperatures   Caffeine timing

Darkness   Limited alcohol

Getting out of bed   Breathing exercises

What You Can Do on Your Own

As you can see, there are many ways you can support your ability to sleep. As you read through these possibilities, choose at least one thing you could start tonight. The earlier you begin, the faster the benefits of a new sleep routine will start to accrue.

Inoculate your bedroom from stress. Your bedroom should be a calming, serene place for relaxation and sleep. Your bed should be a sacred space your body recognizes as a place you go to rest, repair, and connect—not a place you go to worry, work, talk about stressful things, solve murder mysteries, or binge bad TV (or even good TV). Avoid talking on the phone, paying your bills, or scrolling through the news headlines on your phone while you're in this space. If you have a TV or computer in your bedroom, move it to another part of your home and save your bed for sleeping and sex only. If you need the TV to turn off your brain, try using a white noise machine instead, or watch it in another room until you feel ready for bed.

I know that this is not possible in all living spaces, but try to avoid having a desk or treadmill right next to your bed. If you live in a studio apartment, a standing room divider will shield those things from view, or you can even throw a tapestry or sheet over your desk before you go to bed at night.

Routinize your getting-ready-for-bed ritual. You need a bedtime routine to signal to your body that it's time to wind down, just like toddlers do. While a bedtime routine for a kid might be a glass of milk, a bath, a book, and then lights out, yours can be anything that makes you feel cozy and drowsy (and ideally, device-free). Maybe a bath or a shower, a quick journaling or meditation session, or a cup of Sleepytime tea while reading. You already have some kind of bedtime routine that probably involves brushing your teeth and changing into sleep clothes—this just adds a little extra to your already established habit and makes the process a little more intentionally relaxing.

Stick to a consistent schedule. If you have a pet, you know that they know when it's time to eat, to go outside, and to go to bed, even though they don't know how to read a clock. That's because they have an internal clock, and so do you. It's called your circadian rhythm, which is a daily symphony of rising and falling hormones and other chemical messengers orchestrated by the pineal gland in your brain. Your circadian rhythm takes cues from the sun and your daily habits to cue the rise of melatonin in the evening, which makes you sleepy; and cortisol in the morning, which helps you have the energy to face the day. When you stick to a consistent schedule for sleep and waking, your circadian rhythm supports you and makes it easier both to fall asleep and to wake up the next morning. To keep your inner clock running smoothly, on the weekend, try not to go to bed or wake up more than an hour or so of variance from your weekday times. Of course, you'll have to veer from these times occasionally—for travel or other events, or to get up with a sick child or pet—but the more you can honor a regular schedule, the more aligned you'll be to your internal rhythm.

Keep it cool. As mentioned, temperature is always an important component of sleep because our body temperature naturally falls during sleep. This is even more vital during perimenopause, when your internal thermometer starts to go a little haywire and you start running hot at night. During the winter, consider turning the heat down overnight, or turning up the AC in warmer months, so that your sleeping space is about sixty-five degrees or less. You may also want to start sleeping in fewer clothes, using lighter bedding, or taking a more layered approach to your bedding so that you can toss off a blanket or two in the night if you start running hot or use all layers if you get cold. There are also pajamas, pillows, sheets, and mattresses that are designed to help you sleep cooler at night. I love the cooling sheets from Rest.

Keep it dark and quiet. Any light in the blue end of the spectrum that you're exposed to after sunset can disrupt your sleep-wake cycle. Blackout curtains are an investment but they do wonders for promoting restful sleep, especially if there are artificial lights visible from your bedroom windows. Even alarm clocks and power buttons on electronics can be bright enough to disrupt sleep. Look for an alarm clock with red numbers because red light (like firelight) doesn't activate the nervous system. Consider using a sleep mask to block out as much light as possible.

The same goes for noise—you want as few noise interruptions as possible. White noise machines are great for blocking out ambient noises. And if your snoring partner or pet regularly wakes you up, consider ways to minimize your exposure. That could mean sleeping with earplugs or sleeping separately.

Build up your sleep hunger. Here is a counterintuitive, game-changing tip: if you wake up in the middle of the night and don't fall back asleep after about ten minutes, be like Aniyah, and get out of bed and do something that's not too stimulating in another location—try reading (so long as it's not a thriller), meditating, journaling, coloring, or listening to jazz or classical music or a podcast or audio book (just don't get sucked into checking your email or the headlines) or guided relaxation, ideally using a light with an amber bulb so the light doesn't wake you up. What you *don't* want to do is to go anywhere that is brightly lit or do anything that might be considered productive, because both can stimulate wakefulness.

Getting out of bed in the middle of the night may seem like a surefire way to sleep less, but staying in bed tossing and turning reinforces the idea that your bed is not for sleeping, it's a place for worrying. This is also known as sleep restriction—a CBT-I technique that seeks to limit the amount of time you spend in bed when you aren't sleeping so that you begin to spend a larger percentage of the time you are in bed actually asleep.

As long as you aren't doing anything that promotes excitement and wakefulness, your drowsiness—or what sleep scientists call sleep hunger—will continue to build. When you feel sleepy again, come back to bed. You are not going to want to get up, but it's actually faster to get out of bed. In the book *The Alchemy of Us*, Ainissa Ramirez writes that up until the Industrial Revolution, it was common practice for humans to sleep in two different segments of the night, separated by an hour or so of being awake (like the opposite of taking a siesta during the day).[5] Learning this has helped me feel like less of an outlier on those nights I am up for a while in the middle of the night, which helps me stay calm enough to get back to sleep.

If you try getting out of bed and you don't feel your drowsiness build, or you do feel your eyelids get heavy but you don't drift off once you get back in bed, remember that rest is the next best thing to sleep. Get comfortable (preferably in a location other than your bed, like the couch, so that you don't associate the bed with lying awake) and try to let yourself enjoy another sleep podcast or doing some of the CBT-I techniques on pages 104 and 105. And remember: A poor night's sleep is unpleasant but it isn't fatal.

Try magnesium glycinate. The mineral magnesium is a relaxant that can help you drift off to sleep. (It also relaxes the muscles of your digestive tract, meaning it can make you more regular—although it won't make you have to wake up in the middle of the night to go to the bathroom.) Try 300–400 mg a half hour before getting in bed.

Do a little before-bed yoga. Just as babies and toddlers benefit from a regular bedtime routine to help them transition into sleep mode, so do you. Since you already have a bedtime routine, adding another five to ten minutes of some yoga stretches builds in a chance to quiet your mind and release some physical stress. The more relaxed you are, the easier it will be to drift off and the more likely you will be to stay asleep. Science bears this out: A 2019 meta-analysis found that regular yoga practice delivered significant improvements in sleep quality and reduced insomnia severity.[6] The more consistent you can be with your before-bed yoga, the more your body will start to get the cue that it's time to wind down. You may even start to crave that part of your routine.

An easy and relaxing routine is: simple seated twist, cobbler's pose, wide-legged straddle, child's pose, and corpse pose. You can also do an internet search for "bedtime yoga" and get many other routine suggestions. And if yoga's not your thing, that same 2019 meta-analysis saw similar benefit from other mind-body therapies, including meditation, tai chi, and qigong.

Give self-hypnosis a try. Self-hypnosis may sound strange or perhaps even scary, but it simply means getting yourself into a profoundly relaxed state and then consciously focusing your attention on a specific outcome—in this case, falling and staying asleep, although you can also use self-hypnosis for other purposes, such as to set goal-related intentions or to release stress. Although the "self" in "self-hypnosis" suggests that you have to know how to get yourself into a hypnotic state, there are many apps that will talk you through it, and all you have to do is listen and follow along. My favorites are Harmony, HypnoBox, and Digipill. In addition to better sleep, self-hypnosis can help you reduce overall stress levels, which will help you feel better when you're awake, too.

Clean up your caffeine act. There's nothing wrong with having a caffeinated beverage or two in the morning to help you get going, but having caffeine after 2:00 p.m. can interfere with your ability to fall asleep that night. That's because caffeine has a half-life of about six hours. So, if you have a cup at 4:00 p.m., half of that caffeine will still be in your system at 10:00 p.m.—and how well would you expect to sleep if you had a half-cup of coffee right before getting in bed? For some women, caffeine can also trigger hot flashes. Believe me, I love my coffee and never want to give it up, but sleep is too precious to me to justify drinking it in the afternoon or evening. If you've been relying on coffee for a midafternoon pick-me-up, try a little movement instead—a quick walk, a dance session, or a set or two of bodyweight exercises such as squats or jumping jacks can perk you right up. Drinking a glass of water, listening to some upbeat music, or even setting the timer on your phone for a fifteen- to twenty-minute nap are also helpful.

Limit your alcohol consumption. Alcohol is technically a depressant, which means that once you've metabolized it, you may feel more awake. If you're having a glass of wine or two right before bed, it's likely you'll awaken in the middle of the night not feeling sleepy. The Centers for Disease Control advises that women have no more than one drink—that's five ounces of wine, twelve ounces of beer, or one ounce of hard liquor—per day. Be honest about how much you're really drinking, limit it to one serving per day, and have that glass earlier in the night for better sleep. Better yet, skip alcohol altogether, or have it only once or twice per week. (I talk more about the health risks of alcohol in chapter 9.)

Also, alcohol (particularly red wine because of the vasodilatory effects) is another hot flash trigger—yet another reason to be very mindful of your consumption.

There are lots of nonalcoholic wine and beer options out there if you want the feeling of having a cocktail without the actual alcohol. A lot of my patients tell me they will pour themselves some kombucha—a fizzy, fermented tea with different flavors that delivers probiotics, which are good for mental health as well as digestion—in a wine glass. Add a few berries for an extra health kick. A friend of mine buys a tincture of hops—a component of many IPA-style beers that is said by herbalists to have calming properties. She mixes a dropperful of hops in a glass of seltzer to get some of that "taking the edge off" feeling that drinking a beer can provide without the alcohol.

Stimulate the parasympathetic nervous system with breathing exercises. Your autonomic nervous system—which rules all the functions of the body that work without you having to think about them, such as your heart rate, respiration, digestion, and arousal—is broken up into three branches: the sympathetic, the parasympathetic, and the enteric nervous systems. The sympathetic nervous system coordinates the stress response, the parasympathetic runs the rest and digest functions, and the enteric manages how your digestive system metabolizes your food. Typically, our always-on modern lifestyles mean that our sympathetic nervous system is more likely to be activated, which diverts energy away from the parasympathetic realm, where we feel relaxed, at peace, and easily able to succumb to restful sleep.

Although breathing occurs without our conscious effort, when we decide to focus on and influence the breath, we can send a signal to our sympathetic nervous system that it is okay for it to quiet down. This brings our parasympathetic nervous system online, which helps pave the way for sleep, settles the heart rate, and can even help to resolve hot flashes.

Try incorporating just a few minutes of breathing exercises into your nightly wind-down routine. Dim the lights, sit or lie down, and breathe in slowly and evenly for a count of five and out for a count of five. Repeat for one to three minutes. Although it is helpful for sleep, you can do this technique throughout your day to combat stress in the moment and clear your head. Try it after you've eaten lunch, after a meeting, or as you sit in your car at a red light.

What I *Don't* Recommend

I suggest avoiding benzodiazepine medications such as Xanax and Klonopin, and benzo-like sleep meds such as Ambien, because they are addictive and—although the data is mixed—many studies have found a link between their use and an increased risk of dementia.[7] Aside from the addictive nature of these medications, the biggest risk is that they can wipe out your anxiety in a flash or put you to sleep in a few minutes. Which means you don't have to build your relaxation and sleep hygiene muscles. So, while that may sound great, the downside is that in the long term, dealing with your anxiety or putting yourself to sleep gets harder and harder to do, leading to the addiction, or physiological reliance, on these medications.

To be clear, these medications have their place. They are typically prescribed during a time of high need, such as a divorce or the passing of a parent. Benzos reduce your neuronal activity (those swirling thoughts) in minutes, making them helpful for things like panic attacks; airplane travel (if you have a fear of flying); or getting an MRI, which requires you to remain still inside of a very small, enclosed space. The benzo-like meds (such as Ambien and Ativan) take a little longer—up to thirty minutes—and are more sedating. They increase the activity of GABA, which can really knock you out. And yet, if something sounds too good to be true, it generally is. While these medications are intended for short-term use, it's very easy to become dependent on them. In addition to being physiologically addicting, it's also very easy to become psychologically dependent on these meds—making it hard to adopt other practices to self-regulate your anxiety.

If you are already reliant on sleep meds, work with your clinician to slowly wean yourself off them. If you are currently taking 1 mg, you might go down to .5 mg for a period of time, then .25 mg, then perhaps

.25 mg every other day. Because there is often a physiological dependence, it's not advisable to go cold turkey. Getting off sleep or antianxiety meds may sound impossible, but it is doable when you simultaneously create better relaxation and sleep hygiene habits. In my practice, I will often prescribe nightly oral progesterone to help foster drowsiness and relaxation while a patient is in the weaning process. Yet another win for hormone support!

CHAPTER 6

Dragging Yourself Through Life

Allison, a fifty-one-year-old real estate agent, once loved getting up every morning to check the new listings and send updates to her clients, but over the last few months she had come to dread mornings. At our first meeting, Allison told me it seemed like her typical drive had just evaporated. She was embarrassed to admit it, but she no longer cared about making deals or finding her clients their dream homes—the prospect just wasn't as exciting. Allison's son had also recently left for college, and with him gone, the house felt lonely and cold, which was also how she felt. Allison couldn't put her finger exactly on when this happened, and she felt ashamed, saying that she had no reason to feel this way. Her son was thriving, she had a loving partner, they just renovated their kitchen, and together they had purchased their dream beach house. But she couldn't shake the feeling that something wasn't right about how down she felt. When she started avoiding getting together with her friends and family because she didn't want to have to pretend that she felt fine, she knew it was time to seek professional help.

Layla, a thirty-eight-year-old banking executive, had been making mistakes at work. To her it felt like the neurons in her brain just weren't connected, so that whatever she was trying to remember—a particular statistic, or a colleague's name—couldn't make its way to her mouth; these things had all come easily before.

Layla was also waking up a lot in the middle of the night to pee, and now, unlike in her twenties and early thirties, she couldn't just fall back asleep. Her fatigue certainly wasn't helping her memory recall, and she was also struggling to get herself out of bed in the mornings. She hadn't been feeling up to going to the kickboxing classes that she once loved. Layla's primary care doctor suspected fibromyalgia or maybe chronic fatigue syndrome. Unconvinced, she consulted an infectious disease specialist, who thought it could be either long COVID or chronic Lyme disease and was running a battery of tests. More confused than ever, Layla decided to drastically reduce her hours at work, thinking if she just lowered her stress, she'd be able to bounce back. Finally, after her sister suggested that perhaps these symptoms could be related to perimenopause, Layla ended up in my office.

What Layla and Allison both shared was that they felt like they were having to drag themselves through their days with what felt like none of their usual energy or motivation. This particular symptom set can have repercussions that run far and wide through a woman's life. In addition to a greatly diminished quality of life, you may be worrying that you aren't able to perform at your job—which might mean you don't go for that promotion. Or, like Layla, you might cut back your hours, or you switch to a lower-stress, but also lower-paying, job, which can then have financial consequences. In fact, one out of five American women have considered leaving a job due to menopause symptoms, according to a 2023 report.[1] Your relationships with friends and family may also suffer if you don't have the energy to meet up or don't want to share how you're really feeling. Or, maybe you feel disconnected from your partner because you've withdrawn, thinking you don't have anything interesting to share or to give.

But perhaps what's most distressing about this symptom set is the changes in cognition. According to my own research that was published in *Menopause*, the journal of the Menopause Society, the symptom that troubles women the most is brain fog.[2] For all the attention that hot flashes receive from media and researchers, and as inconvenient and unpleasant as they can be, I have found that to my patients, nothing is as disruptive as the cognitive changes that are linked to the decline of estrogen levels. I'll cover more about estrogen's impact on the brain later in this chapter, but for now, I want you to know that brain fog is not forever. The brain is amazingly adaptable—the technical term for this ability is "neuroplasticity." In perimenopause, the brain is going through a rewiring process to learn how to operate with less estrogen, and it will come back online eventually. But when you are in the thick of it, brain fog can be downright scary—especially as we women are known for our ability to keep track of multiple things in our heads at all times, while also managing our personal and professional lives.

As we covered in chapter 1, estrogen is so important to every organ system and at the cellular level that as we start to lose it, we may experience widespread effects. One of the reasons perimenopause is often so challenging is because it can be a bit of a chameleon, producing symptoms that could be attributable to any number of other conditions. For this symptom set, the possible other causes for the fatigue, malaise, fuzzy thinking, and loss of joie de vivre align with the descriptions of so many other health concerns, from depression to Alzheimer's. Because perimenopause isn't on a lot of our individual radars, and since so many doctors have not been trained in it, it doesn't often appear on a list of these possible causes. Which means that many women with this symptom set will be misdiagnosed as having depression, low thyroid function, chronic fatigue syndrome, fibromyalgia or some other autoimmune condition, or a rare infectious disease.

The problems here are twofold: (1) Misdiagnosis leads to mismanagement. Mismanagement likely means your symptoms will continue while you begin experiencing new symptoms that are the side effects of the treatment for your misdiagnosis. I have seen many women prescribed medications for low thyroid function or even given steroids for unlikely autoimmune conditions that make them feel worse. Meanwhile, the true cause of the primary symptoms remains unaddressed. And (2), many of these misdiagnoses come with a stigma, when what's really going on is a basic, universal physiological process. And that can make you feel worse about yourself and experience more stress and anxiety than if you were simply told your symptoms could very well be linked to perimenopause.

DRAGGING YOURSELF THROUGH LIFE AT A GLANCE

Symptoms:

- Brain fog
- Low energy
- Low motivation
- Difficulty feeling joy and purpose
- Urinary symptoms (waking up to pee, UTIs, urinary incontinence)

Causative factors:

Declining estrogen

The Difference Between Early-Onset Alzheimer's and Perimenopausal Brain Fog

Early-onset Alzheimer's is a form of dementia that starts before the age of sixty-five, most often in the forties or fifties. It is also highly genetic, and the genetic mutation thought to be the cause is extremely rare—only a few hundred people have it.[3]

That being said, dementia is something every woman should have on her radar, because at this point, the odds are that one in five women will develop it in their lifetime.[4] And although the disease generally doesn't present until after age sixty-five, it is slow to develop, meaning that brain changes can start as early as our forties, just as we are losing our reproductive hormones.

Walking into a room and forgetting why you're there, having trouble recalling a word or someone's name, or misplacing your phone are all very typical scenarios for perimenopause-related brain fog. What isn't typical is getting lost in familiar surroundings, asking the same questions again and again, or having difficulty doing familiar tasks, like paying bills.

Even though the stats on women and Alzheimer's are concerning, what's heartening is that science is beginning to understand that there is much we can do to prevent dementia—including getting regular exercise, keeping alcohol consumption moderate or minimal, not smoking, and maintaining robust social connections. According to the *Lancet*, one of the oldest and most prestigious medical journals, 45 percent of dementia cases are preventable.[5] While science isn't settled on whether hormone therapy can prevent dementia, a 2023 meta-analysis of fifty-one studies found that women who started on HT in their forties or fifties and stayed on it for at least ten years saw a 26 percent reduction in dementia risk.[6]

Motherhood and Perimenopause: A Potent Mix

Let me begin this section by saying: If you're not a mother, whether by choice or by circumstance, I respect your choices and empathize with any of your losses. I understand you may want to skip right over this section, but if you have friends or family members stressed out by motherhood, you might share some of these insights with them and help them to understand what they're dealing with.

No matter how old your kids are when you hit perimenopause, your shifting hormones may make motherhood feel extra hard. If you had kids in your mid- to late thirties or in your forties, you could experience a pretty big decline in hormones after birth and breastfeeding that could make sleep even more difficult, your energy levels feel even lower, and perhaps cause your mood to drop in a way that resembles postpartum depression. If your kids are school-age when you develop symptoms, declining hormones may make you feel like your irritability is peaking as your patience is bottoming out, and brain fog might make juggling the many tasks of raising kids feel more challenging. If you've got a tween or young teenage daughter, you could be dealing with both perimenopause and puberty under one roof—which, I can tell you from experience, is no joke! If your kids are in their late teens and leaving home soon, your hormonal reality could make the lessening of your daily parental duties feel like your purpose is also leaving the nest and intensify feelings of grief. You may also no longer have reasons to multitask, which is essentially a high-stakes brain game that you engaged in nearly every day when your kids were home, and that absence can contribute to feeling that you're losing your mental sharpness.

However old your kids are, perimenopause symptoms could make you feel like you're a bad mom (yelling at your kids or not wanting to engage in the usual family activities) or that you are having an unusually hard time with motherhood. I also know that the symptoms of perimenopause impact women's quality of life in all areas, including in our role as mothers, and as romantic partners as well. My patients confide in me that they feel disconnected from their spouse because they're on a journey their spouse can't possibly understand, or that they're so irritable that they are picking fights, or they don't feel like having sex, or all of the above, and it's causing stress in their marriage or partnership. I'm pointing out these connections to raise your awareness of the possible troublesome tentacles perimenopause may be extending into other parts of your life.

It's our tendency as women to brush uncomfortable feelings away and say we're too busy to take better care of ourselves. We may be motivated by taking care of other people and put ourselves on the back burner. If that sounds like you, perhaps thinking of how your symptoms may be impacting the people you love in addition to how they affect you directly can clarify why it really is worth the time and energy it will take to schedule an appointment with your provider, or find a new clinician if yours isn't particularly helpful. Yes, it's a pain, but you are precious all on your own, *and* you are important to a lot of other people. Remember, perimenopause can last up to ten years, and once you're in menopause, your symptoms can continue for another several years. Your well-being is too important to wait.

Brain Fog and Depression—a Double Whammy

If you've been feeling like your brain isn't working the way it used to, you're likely right. As we've learned, the brain is filled with estrogen receptors, particularly the parts of the brain that help us regulate our emotions, store information in our short-term memory so that we can access it easily, and pay attention for prolonged periods of time. So, is it any wonder, then, that it can feel like our emotions are all over the place, we can't remember why we walked into a room, and we're generally scattered? In addition, estrogen is an anti-inflammatory, and as it declines we can experience more neuroinflammation, which often plays a role in migraines and other short-term cognitive changes.

I've learned a lot from neuroscientist Dr. Lisa Mosconi, author of *The Menopause Brain*. Through her studies, which involve brain imaging of women before and after menopause, she has discovered that the amount of energy in the brain changes significantly over the course of perimenopause. Premenopause, a woman's brain scan lights up in a way that resembles an aerial view of a major metropolitan area at night. Postmenopause, that same woman's brain has illumination equivalent to the bird's-eye view of a small suburb at best, demonstrating the redistribution of brain function as estrogen declines through this transition. Yet the news isn't all bad. Dr. Mosconi also shares that there are multiple aspects of brain function that improve during the hormonal transition. We become less likely to have big emotional responses, and we are better able to reframe things in a positive way. We also have an easier time accessing empathy (instead of judgment of others). And—this is a biggie—Dr. Mosconi also reports that women are happier in postmenopause. Not just happier in general, but happier than they were premenopause. Multiple things contribute to this postmenopause uptick—being done with the inconvenience of periods, no PMS, and not having to worry about contraception chief among them. It's also the dawn of an entirely new life stage—one where you may be able to put your needs, desires, and curiosity at the top of the list, for maybe the first time in a very long time. So, there is light at the end of the tunnel. I know this information may not actually help you think more clearly or feel happier *right now*, but I do think it's helpful to know that the way you're currently feeling isn't permanent. It's certainly helpful to know you can take an active role to feel better, mentally and cognitively, in your current reality. When it comes to brain fog and feeling blah, you don't have to wait it out.

Perimenopause's Effects on Autoimmune Conditions

If you have an autoimmune condition, such as rheumatoid arthritis, Hashimoto's disease, lupus, celiac disease, chronic fatigue syndrome, or Sjögren's syndrome, it can be easy to confuse perimenopause symptoms with a flare, especially because you are likely more finely attuned to those symptoms than you are to perimenopause. When your reproductive hormones start to shift, that can either introduce new symptoms or appear to worsen existing symptoms.

Just because you have an autoimmune condition does not mean you can't treat your perimenopause symptoms. There are no medications for autoimmunity that you can't use with hormone therapy. It will be essential to work with a trained health-care provider in your life who is monitoring your dosages and your symptoms for you.

Finally, it's helpful to track all of your symptoms to see if what might be a flare from one of your chronic conditions has a cyclical component (even if that cycle is erratic), and to assess what kinds of impact any perimenopausal treatments you start may have. Perhaps hormones were actually the cause of some of what appeared to be flares, and the hope is that HT will bring some relief.

DISCERNING THE DIFFERENCE BETWEEN PERIMENOPAUSE AND HYPOTHYROIDISM

Perimenopause and hypothyroidism—an underactive thyroid—share many symptoms, including low energy, weight gain, fatigue, irregular periods, drier skin, changes in sexual function and desire, and mood changes. If perimenopause isn't on your radar, and you're experiencing these symptoms, you may assume it's probably because your thyroid is sluggish. Definitely speak with your doctor about your symptoms and ask to have your thyroid checked just to rule it out. (Low levels of thyroid hormone are fairly easy to treat with the synthetic thyroid hormone Synthroid.) Remember, however, even though women are ten times more likely to have low thyroid than men, only about 5 percent of the US population has hypothyroidism, while nearly every person born with ovaries will experience perimenopause. Statistically speaking, it's more likely to be your reproductive hormones that are triggering your symptoms.

If you already know that you have hypothyroidism, you may find that you need to change your dosage of Synthroid—perhaps even more than once—as you move through perimenopause, because estrogen influences the thyroid, and as it becomes volatile, your levels of thyroid hormone can fluctuate, too.

Helpful Treatments (in the Order I Typically Recommend Them)

For patients who report these symptoms, the labs I recommend are: vitamin D; thyroid panel; iron studies and ferritin; a complete metabolic panel; plus hemoglobin A1C (a measure of your average glucose levels over the last three months); as well as levels of follicle-stimulating hormone (FSH) and testosterone so we can start to clock the decline of these hormones through the perimenopause transition. I also check blood pressure and make sure they're up-to-date with all their screenings, such as mammograms, colonoscopies, and Pap smears.

Once we have these results in hand and can rule out things like low vitamin D or iron levels, or thyroid hormone deficiency, we'll talk through the medical treatments that are typically helpful in treating these symptoms.

Supplemental Estrogen

Because declining estrogen is typically at the root of this cluster of symptoms, I like to try adding FDA-approved estradiol if the patient is a candidate for hormone therapy—whether as a pill, patch, spray, or systemic vaginal ring—to see if symptoms improve, and if so, by how much. The dosage will vary based on a patient's health history, stage of perimenopause, and tolerance. Breast tenderness and increased or excessive bleeding are signs that the dosage is too high.

Although it is true that postmenopausally, it's not recommended to take estrogen on its own without progesterone (because progesterone prevents the uterine lining from building up and reduces the risk of developing uterine cancer later in life), in perimenopause it is okay to use estrogen alone for a period of several months if a woman is still having periods so that we can be sure it's helping the symptom set (we learned this in the previous chapter). If estradiol does help your symptoms and you want to remain on it, you should add progesterone after about six months if you have a uterus (remember, if you have an IUD, you already have the progesterone component of the hormone therapy regimen).

One of my patients, Jamie, is forty-four and has been a mortgage lender for fifteen years. She noticed her brain fog right away when she started having difficulty calculating the numerical versions of different fractions—calculations she'd been doing every day for over a decade. When she started forgetting the names of brokers with whom she regularly did business, she started worrying she could no longer do her job effectively. She became extremely self-conscious about making a glaring mistake. When she started to track her symptoms, we noticed her brain fog was much worse in the luteal phase of her cycle, when estrogen was naturally declining. So we opted for an estradiol patch, which she wears the last two weeks of her cycle, and her facility with numbers and name recall came right back online.

Vaginal Estrogen

Because the vagina and urinary tract have the highest concentration of estrogen receptors in the body, when estrogen starts to decline, these tissues are often some of the first to change—a lack of moisture and an increase in the pH balance (during your reproductive years, an acidic pH of around 5 keeps bacteria at bay; as estrogen declines, pH can rise as high as 6 or 7 and become basic) come first, followed by thinning of the tissues. In addition to painful sex, this can lead to urinary changes, whether that's needing to wake up to pee more often, or even some urinary incontinence, such as leaking a little urine when you sneeze, jump, or cough. Vaginal estrogen is so effective at maintaining the structure and function of these tissues and so very low-risk—I wish it could be sold over-the-counter. For the time being, you do need a prescription from a clinician.

This was the first step for Layla, whom you met at the start of this chapter. She decided to take a vaginal estrogen product because her nighttime awakenings to use the bathroom were resulting in a lot of lost sleep and the fatigue and fuzzy thinking that come with it. It did help her sleep through the night, which then helped with her focus. But when she was still struggling to feel joy and return to the activities she once enjoyed, I suggested she add cognitive behavioral therapy. Devoting that time to talking through her thoughts and feelings helped Layla realize that she wanted to go back to school and switch careers to something that makes her happier. She earned a degree in nonprofit administration and is now teaching financial literacy to underserved populations.

Dopamine Agonists

There is a class of medications that work by amplifying the presence of dopamine—a neurotransmitter that promotes feelings of pleasure and reward, and thus can help with motivation, too. Again, I may be biased, but I like to try FDA-approved estradiol first. I'll move on to these other options if the patient has any contraindications to HT, or if we tried it and it didn't work as well as my patient and I had hoped it would. The two dopamine agonists I recommend are the antidepressant Wellbutrin (bupropion) and a newer medication called Addyi (flibanserin), which has FDA approval to treat reduced sexual desire in premenopausal women by increasing the dopamine level in the brain and helping you feel joy and contentment again—and help bring your libido back, too (because if you're having difficulty feeling pleasure, you're probably not going to want to have sex; I'll be talking more specifically about low libido in chapter 7). Addyi also balances norepinephrine, a neurotransmitter that helps us feel awake, alert, and ready to pay attention. Both Wellbutrin and Addyi can also help with fatigue and feeling blah as well as improve cognition because dopamine acts like a stimulant and gives you a little bit of energy and the ability to maintain your focus.

Allison, the real estate agent you met at the start of this chapter, opted to try Wellbutrin, because she felt and I agreed that her feelings of sadness and lack of purpose were her most troubling symptoms. I also talked with her about the importance of social connection, getting outside, and moving her body (three things I cover in the "What You Can Do on Your Own" section; see page 127), so she added in a Sunday morning walk with a friend to tick all those boxes in one activity. She also started drinking her morning coffee on the porch when the weather cooperated and stretching for a few minutes before bed—all of which helped with her mood and put the pep back in her step.

Continuous Combined Birth Control Pills

Going on birth control pills—and taking them continuously so that you skip the week of placebo pills and go right into the next pack after twenty-one days, or using the NuvaRing or a transdermal patch so that you don't have to remember to take a pill every day—will increase your levels of synthetic estrogen and progesterone. As a reminder, these birth control methods work by stopping the surge of luteinizing hormone (LH) that tells the ovaries to release an egg. The result is that your hormone levels stay steady throughout the month and can help to make you feel more even-keeled, and by extension like you have more energy.

As a bonus, birth control methods can also stop your bleeding, which, although it may not be your primary symptom, can make your life a little less complicated. And, of course, they provide contraception, too, as, otherwise, it is still possible to get pregnant in perimenopause.

I have seen a lot of migraine patients do well on continuous birth control, as hormone volatility can often be a trigger for the onset of migraines. If you suspect you have chronic fatigue syndrome, fibromyalgia, or another autoimmune condition, taking continuous birth control pills can help you and your clinician determine how much your hormone shifts may or may not be contributing to another underlying problem.

Therapy

If you are feeling low, talking to a mental health professional could help support you during this transitional time. As you know, I believe cognitive behavioral therapy (CBT) is a powerful tool for changing your mindset and habits and patterns, but any type of psychological therapy with a trained professional that makes you feel better is a plus.

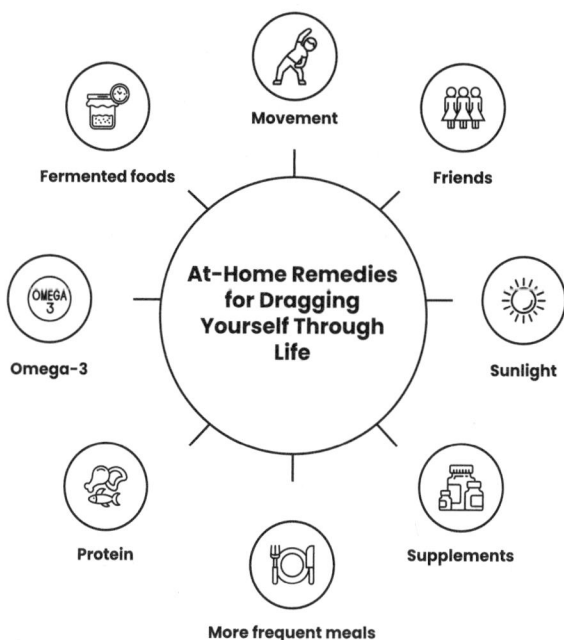

At-Home Remedies for Dragging Yourself Through Life: Movement, Fermented foods, Friends, Omega-3, Sunlight, Protein, More frequent meals, Supplements

What You Can Do on Your Own

Get more movement. I know it can seem cruel to suggest exercise when you may not even feel like getting out of bed, but there is so much data to show that exercise helps boost mood, produces natural painkilling molecules, such as endorphins, and lubricates your joints. If all you can manage is a short walk most days, that's still an accomplishment. If you're able and interested in the possibility, try short, high-intensity interval workouts or weight training or both, as these have been shown to benefit the brain as well as the muscles and the heart. You may need to drag yourself to the gym or down the sidewalk, and you may feel like you're just going through the motions at first, but that will improve as you get going—trust me, I have been there myself. After you are finished, really sit in the feeling of how fun and important and meaningful that was, and that will make it 10 percent easier to get to the next class. If you can, get your exercise outside, preferably in a natural setting like a park or the woods, but even if you're in the middle of the city, the fresh air, natural sunlight, and a view of the sky will up the benefit.

Prioritize time with friends. There's so much good science around the benefits of community. A Harvard study that followed a cohort of people beginning in 1936—the longest longitudinal study ever—found that having good relationships is a huge predictor of both health and happiness.[7] The catch is, you have to actively spend time nurturing those relationships.

If you've had children, you could be coming out of several years where you've felt like most of your attention and energy has gone to your nuclear family and perhaps your friendships have had to take a back burner. That is completely natural and understandable. With three kids under eight, I can identify. Maintaining my relationships is something I constantly have to remind myself to do, and every time I connect with a friend, whether through a text or a DM or in person, I am so thankful that I took the time because it feels so good to reconnect.

Regardless of your parenting status, even though the COVID-19 pandemic was several years ago now, we're still feeling the effects of the ways our lives changed. In 2023, the US surgeon general declared that we have collectively been living through a secondary epidemic of loneliness and isolation.[8] That loneliness has a cost—in physical terms, it raises our risk of premature death by 60 percent, dementia by 50 percent, and heart disease by nearly a third. People who report being lonely are also twice as likely to experience depression than people who never or rarely feel lonely.

All this is to say, put dinner with friends (or a workout—whether it's pickleball, a dance class, a walk, or hitting the gym) on the calendar. As with exercise, you may have to use a decent amount of willpower to propel yourself out the door, but you're going to feel so good during and especially afterward. Even quick gestures, like texting someone when you think of them, count. Whatever you can do to nurture a sense of connection will help you feel more supported and like you're part of a bigger world than whatever's happening within the four walls of your home.

If you are feeling like you aren't in the best place friends-wise, remember that someone doesn't have to be your ride-or-die best friend forever for that relationship to be meaningful to both of you. Researchers have found that so-called weak ties—a terrible name (I think) that refers to people whom you perhaps know only very casually, like the barista at your regular coffee shop, or your neighbor whose dog you say hello to whenever they walk past your house—are very important for happiness and overall well-being.[9] Seminal research on weak ties from the 1970s has found that casual ties to other people are more helpful in getting a job than closer relationships, such as best friends or family members.[10] That's because those so-called weak ties connect you to other social networks and help ensure that you don't get siloed in talking to the same people over and over again.

Another way to kill two birds with one stone is to check out a menopause retreat—essentially a girls' trip you can either take with an existing friend and deepen your relationship or go alone and make new friends while you're there and learning how to care for yourself at this pivotal time in life. These retreats vary from a few hours to a whole day or weekend or even a cruise around the world (like Dr. Mary Claire Haver's the 'Pause Life Retreat, a five-day cruise through the Caribbean. I appeared as a presenter, and the trip was as good for my soul as it was for my mind and body).

Soak up some sunlight. I don't mean tanning—I mean exposing yourself to natural light in the mornings for about ten minutes. Seasonal affective disorder (SAD) is real, and making sure you get morning light exposure can help keep it at bay. This also will help regulate your body's internal clock and circadian rhythm, which means it will help you feel sleepy at night and awake in the morning. If it's just not possible for you to get outside for ten minutes in the morning (although, would it be possible for you to take your morning cup of coffee outdoors?), you can use a blue light device. Designed to ward off SAD, this is a light you can turn on and then set a timer for fifteen to twenty minutes—you can use the light in the bathroom while you're getting ready or at your desk while you're checking email.

Try some strategic supplements. Vitamin B_{12} is great for energy, and since it is naturally highest in animal products, if you are a vegetarian or a vegan, you are at risk of running low. (Nutritional yeast is a good source of B_{12}—it has a vaguely cheesy taste, which makes it great for sprinkling on popcorn.) If your iron levels are low because you're also bleeding more frequently or heavily than usual, an iron supplement may also help (it's best to get tested with the help of your clinician to determine if you actually need more iron). And nearly everyone can use more vitamin D, especially in the winter and spring when you haven't been outdoors much (your body manufactures vitamin D when your skin is exposed to sunlight). Low vitamin D levels (defined as anything under 30 ng/mL) can present as fatigue and mood changes—in other words, the very things that define this symptom set. Vitamin D is super easy to replace—aim for 1,000–2,000 international units (IUs) a day. As for herbs, rhodiola is helpful for relieving stress, anxiety, headache, and depression. And Asian ginseng has long been hailed for boosting energy, mood, and mental performance.

Prioritize protein. Many amino acids present in protein-rich foods play an important role in mental health via supporting the production of neurotransmitters such as serotonin, dopamine, and acetylcholine. Foods such as whole soy products, turkey, chicken, fatty fish, eggs, beans, nuts, and quinoa are excellent sources of protein, and you should be getting 25 grams of protein at every meal. Make sure you're not over-eating refined carbs like bread, pasta, and cereal, which can cause blood sugar spikes and subsequent crashes.

Keep your blood sugar steady. Going long periods of time without eating—whether you're intermittently fasting or so busy you forget to eat—isn't great for sustained energy. If dragging yourself through life is your primary symptom set, aim for eating three meals a day. They should be a protein-rich with plenty of healthy fats (like salmon, avocado, and olive oil) and fiber-rich whole grains (like quinoa, brown rice, or oatmeal) to keep your blood sugar steady. You don't need to add "hangry" to your list of symptoms.

Get plenty of omega-3s. Omega-3 fatty acids are linked to better brain health, and people who regularly eat fish (fatty fish, such as salmon, are rich in omega-3s) and walnuts (also a source of omega-3s) report lower incidences of depression.[11] You can also take an omega-3 fatty acid supplement, between 1,000 and 2,000 mg per day—such as those by Nordic Naturals, which has high purity standards (some fish used for supplements are contaminated with mercury).

Add fermented foods or a probiotic supplement. Your good gut bacteria manufacture neurotransmitters such as serotonin.[12] Nurture this population by eating some fermented foods—such as sauerkraut, miso, unsweetened kefir or yogurt, or kimchi—every day. Instead, or also, you can take a probiotic supplement—the type that needs to be refrigerated, which indicates that the cultures are living. Look to get at least 1 billion and up to 10 billion colony-forming units (CFUs) per day.

CHAPTER 7

Feeling Unrecognizable to Yourself

A few years ago, Helen, a forty-eight-year-old English professor, scheduled an appointment with me because she'd been feeling off. As she put it, "It's like I woke up on my forty-eighth birthday a completely different person."

It started one night when Helen woke up soaked in sweat. At first, she thought she must have the flu. She canceled her classes for that day and stayed home, but the fever never came. She went back to work the next day and chalked it up to a fluke, but a few days later, those night sweats came roaring back. Soon it wasn't just at night—she'd been breaking out in a sweat at random times during the day, too. Helen told me that even though she doesn't like to bare her arms in the classroom, she's been forced to wear sleeveless tops under all her blazers so she can whip her jacket off whenever a hot flash comes on.

Helen wondered if it could be long COVID—she had caught the virus just before her birthday and had heard about potentially long-lasting effects. But there was more going on than just the sweating.

Helen's naturally curly hair had morphed into frizz. In addition to this change in texture, her long hair contributed to her general sense of being overheated, so she had recently cut it short.

Between feeling achy in the mornings and the way her low back acted up whenever she sat at her desk for prolonged periods, she started to wonder if she might have an autoimmune condition—at least that's what the articles she found on the internet suggested. Those anxious late-night internet searches were cutting into her sleep, and the stress and fatigue they resulted in weren't helping, either.

Helen also noticed that sex had started to feel different. It seemed that it was getting harder and harder to have an orgasm, and sometimes sex was even downright painful.

Overall, Helen felt like something had taken over her body—it seemed like even her body odor had changed. And perhaps most disturbing, she was forgetting things. Her husband started lightly teasing her that every time she left the house, she'd come back two minutes later because she'd left something important behind. It was inconvenient at home, but when she had trouble recalling the name of the author whose book she was discussing with her students, it was worrisome.

At her most recent primary care appointment, Helen had brought up her various symptoms. Her doctor suggested that Helen needed to reduce her stress so that she could focus better and enjoy sex more. She was also told that her labs "were normal," which made her feel like her concerns were all in her head. Helen felt hopeless as she walked out of that appointment, but the next day, she was motivated to get some clarity on what was going on with her.

Helen remembered seeing a few posts on social media listing the symptoms of perimenopause, but she hadn't read them too closely, thinking perimenopause was for women in their fifties. That day, she searched "symptoms of perimenopause" online, and the results she found connected everything she was experiencing—the hair changes, new body odor, painful sex, brain fog, and hot flashes—into one diagnosis that made perfect sense. One more Google search for "perimenopause doctor" led her to my office.

When Helen came to see me, we talked through all of her symptoms and prioritized which ones she wanted to target first. Since heavy bleeding wasn't something she was dealing with (her periods were coming at erratic intervals, but they weren't particularly heavy), we decided to try two forms of estrogen—local vaginal estrogen to ease her discomfort during sex, and a low-dose systemic estrogen gel to use daily in the morning to address her hot flashes. (If you're experiencing heavy bleeding, estrogen can initially make it worse; so it's best to address your bleeding first, as we covered in chapter 4, before considering estrogen.)

Within a couple of weeks, her hot flashes were greatly reduced, in both frequency and intensity, which meant she was sleeping better, which also meant her brain fog had started to clear. After a few months, sex wasn't painful anymore, although Helen admitted she still really didn't feel like having it, and she missed that closeness with her husband and the stress relief it provided. Because of that, we next added in a testosterone gel, which, as you'll learn, is a way to treat low sexual desire in perimenopausal women.

By the time her forty-ninth birthday came around, Helen felt like she had a new lease on life. She wasn't exactly back to her old self—she kept her short haircut, for example, because she loved both how it looked and how easy it was to style—but she was feeling confident in her body and about moving into the next phase of her life.

**FEELING UNRECOGNIZABLE TO YOURSELF
SYMPTOM SET AT A GLANCE**

Symptoms:

- Hot flashes and night sweats
- Low libido
- Brain fog
- Physical aches and pains
- Sudden change in how you're feeling and acting

Underlying causes:

- Declining estrogen
- Declining progesterone
- Declining testosterone

If you experience the "Feeling Unrecognizable to Yourself" symptom set, it often seems that you feel very different, very quickly, like all parts of your body decided to go on strike at once. I've had many women sit across from me at my desk and tell me that they feel like they don't even recognize themselves in the mirror, as changes to hair, skin, body shape, and yes, even body odor, can occur during the perimenopausal transition, and things that they used to enjoy or be good at, like decorating for the holidays, remembering a long to-do list, or even having sex, suddenly go out the window. I commonly hear things like "Dr. Hirsch, I don't want to be touched ever again." I also hear from women that they rely on their calendar and their Notes app to remember everything, and as a result of this loss of confidence, they're not speaking up as much at work or at home. It's typically a big shift from baseline that happens over what feels like just a few months, and it can be so overwhelming to some women that they feel like their entire personality has changed. Many different things are happening because all three of your primary reproductive hormones—estrogen, progesterone, and testosterone—are declining at the same time. At some point, those lowering levels reach a tipping point where multiple symptoms manifest at once.

Since this symptom set is so broad, I'm splitting the rest of this chapter into two sections: (1) information on treating hot flashes and brain fog; and (2) information on addressing low libido.

Treatments That Can Help with Hot Flashes and Brain Fog (in the Order I Typically Recommend Them)

When patients come to me with a suite of symptoms that fit the "Feeling Unrecognizable to Yourself" type, the lab tests I'll generally order include a hormone panel to look at levels of estrogen and testosterone—even though these tests capture only one day and aren't all that insightful, they can be helpful in establishing a baseline and determining if low testosterone might be a factor if low libido is present. I'll also order a thyroid panel to check if hypothyroidism might be behind the fatigue and brain fog.

Because this symptom set is so wide-ranging and nonspecific, I'll also want to rule out other possible contributing conditions such as diabetes and autoimmunity. To help do that, I'll test levels of C-reactive protein (CRP, which is a nonspecific inflammatory marker that might suggest an autoimmune condition if it comes back elevated); a chemistry panel (that checks kidney and liver function, to rule out fatty liver and kidney dysfunction, as well as pancreatitis); hemoglobin A1C (to test for diabetes); and a metabolic panel and complete blood count, just to make sure there's no rumblings of something deeper, such as cardiovascular disease. Very often, these labs come back not showing any other obvious cause, which is helpful because it points that much more strongly toward perimenopause as the primary underlying physiological factor, and we have proven tools for addressing hormonal changes. Let's look at what those are.

Hormone Therapy

Since all three hormones are contributing to this symptom set, generally, all three hormones can help when taken as combined HT. However, I advise against starting all three at once (and of course, talk with your clinician about your symptoms, your priorities, your quality of life, and your health history to determine which HT route suits you best). Generally, we start with one form of HT and add on another component after four to six weeks. Which one you begin with depends in large part on which symptom is causing you the most angst. If it's low libido, that points toward starting with testosterone. If it's hot flashes, night sweats, or painful sex, I would likely recommend starting with estradiol. And if it's mood changes, difficulty relaxing, and a lack of sleep, I'd recommend starting with progesterone.

If you've been wondering if you might be dealing with something either infectious, like long COVID, or autoimmune-related, like chronic fatigue, trying HT can help rule out those other concerns. If taking hormones helps your symptoms resolve, that strongly suggests the root of the problem was hormonal in nature.

A TOUR THROUGH THE ESTROGEN THERAPY OPTIONS

Here's a quick guide to the various types of estrogen.

Transdermal patch: An estradiol patch lasts either three and a half days or seven days. It's a sticker about the size of two quarters that you wear on your low abdomen. Some patches— including the CombiPatch or Climara Pro—combine estradiol with progesterone.

What I like about the patch is that you only need to think about it once or twice a week. What some women don't love is that the patch can be mildly irritating to their skin. The adhesive is remarkably strong—which is a good thing— but this also means it can accumulate a ring of unsightly gunk that is hard to remove and may rub off on your underwear. If you take a nightly bath, or do hot yoga, or just find that it doesn't stick very well, the patch may also come off. Some women find that they notice the benefit of estrogen wearing off on the last day or two of each patch's life, only to come back in a rush when they apply a new patch (I call this the "whooshing effect," although it is typically only a factor with a patch that you change once a week, not the biweekly patch). While many women do great on the patch, if you experience any of these downsides, a gel, spray, or pill may be a better fit.

Transdermal gel or spray: Estradiol gels are applied every day to your inner thigh; the spray is administered to your forearm. While you have to remember to apply them daily, the gel and spray have a more consistent dose than the patch, less skin irritation, and no annoying ring of gunk.

Oral pills: If you aren't taking a lot of medications and don't have a history of hypertension, diabetes, high cholesterol, or migraines, there is also the option to take a daily oral pill. (This is the form that I take. I find it to be the easiest, but I took birth control for years and it is second nature at this point.)

I mention these conditions as limiting factors for oral estradiol because taking it orally does come with a very low increased risk of developing an unprovoked blood clot. One to two women out of one thousand who are postmenopausal and not taking HT will develop a blood clot. For postmenopausal women who take oral estrogen, that risk rises to two to four women out of one thousand. Transdermal estrogen does not increase the baseline risk of one to two women out of a thousand. For reference, the risk of a blood clot on HT is still lower than the risk of a blood clot on oral birth control.[1]

Vaginal ring: And finally, the Femring releases systemic estrogen over three months, and you can change it on your own (no appointments to get it replaced). This is the most set-it-and-forget-it option, at least until the four times a year you need to replace it.

Nonhormonal Options

If you're looking for a nonhormonal option to help with the vasomotor symptoms (hot flashes and night sweats), you have options, including:

- **Fezolinetant (Veozah)**, a nonhormonal daily pill that is FDA-approved to reduce hot flashes, can be a great option if you aren't a good candidate for hormone therapy. It works by binding to estrogen receptors in the part of the brain that regulates body temperature, which helps you not break out into a huge sweat at the slightest change in ambient temperature. Veozah really only helps with hot flashes, not hot flashes and a handful of other symptoms, like systemic estrogen. At the time of this writing, there are no generic versions of Veozah, which means the price is pretty high—nearly $600 for a thirty-day supply, although your pharmacist may be able to help you find a coupon that lowers the cost. (See "Appendix A: Frequently Asked Questions" in the back of the book for additional information on Veozah.)

- **Wellbutrin (bupropion)**, the dopamine agonist that I also mentioned as a treatment for the "Dragging Yourself Through Life" symptom set, and that we'll learn more about in the next chapter, "Gaining Weight for No (Apparent) Reason," can help with focus, energy, and fatigue.

- **Brisdelle (paroxetine salt)** is a nonhormonal selective serotonin reuptake inhibitor (SSRI) that has FDA approval to treat hot flashes. (Remember, serotonin and estrogen like to be together, so when you boost serotonin, you also tend to increase estrogen.) Brisdelle is the same medication as Paxil, just at a lower dose.

- **Supplements:** Some supplements can also support estrogen levels and provide some relief, to varying degrees, of low-estrogen symptoms such as hot flashes and night sweats, including:

  - **Supplements containing phytoestrogens,** which are naturally occurring chemicals in plants, such as soy and flaxseed, that mimic the effects of estrogen in the body. Two such supplements are Equelle, which contains soy isoflavones; and Estroven, which contains black cohosh, isoflavones, and rhapontic rhubarb extract.

  - **Ashwagandha,** an herbal supplement that has been found to reduce the symptoms of perimenopause that negatively impact quality of life and even boost estrogen levels when taken twice daily (300 mg) for eight weeks.[2]

  - **Black cohosh.** There's good evidence to support this herbal remedy, which can reduce the frequency and severity of hot flashes by binding to estrogen receptors—also taken twice a day (40 mg) for eight weeks.[3]

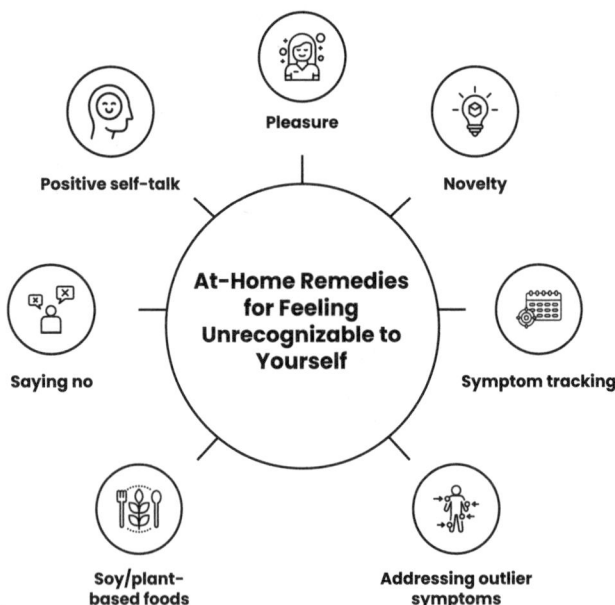

Pleasure

Positive self-talk

Novelty

At-Home Remedies for Feeling Unrecognizable to Yourself

Saying no

Symptom tracking

Soy/plant-based foods

Addressing outlier symptoms

What You Can Do on Your Own to Feel More Like Yourself

Move a little more. At the risk of sounding like a broken record, exercise has many wide-ranging benefits that can help you find your groove again. While I believe that every perimenopausal woman benefits from strength-training (which I discuss in both chapters 8 and 9), for this symptom set, I'm not even talking about "fitness." You don't have to break a sweat or find a half hour or more; you just need to do something to get your body moving. A quick walk when you can. A little bit of stretching before bed or while you watch TV. Ten minutes of yoga after you get home from work. You just want to get your blood flowing a little more (increased circulation means more oxygen and more energy throughout your body, including your brain and your sexual organs), give your muscles a chance to get a little looser, and bring your awareness into your body and away from your thoughts as often as you can manage. It will help lessen your experience of stress, reset your mind, and give your mood a little boost. If you're inspired to grab some weights now, don't let me stop you! But if you need a more gradual entry into the world of exercise that is totally fine, and still totally helpful.

Do things just for the pleasure of it. Play music while you're cooking dinner—maybe music you used to love in high school or college that will get you nodding your head, singing along, or outright dancing. I get a lot of joy from reading; my genre of the moment is what my husband jokingly calls fairy smut but is technically called "romantasy," such as *Fourth Wing* by Rebecca Yarros or *A Court of Thorns and Roses* by Sarah J. Maas. Call your friends, or better yet, make a date to get together with a friend. These relationships are powerful; they remind us of who we are and inspire us to think about all the things we could be.

Invite novelty into your life. While many of my patients say they want to feel like themselves again—and I understand and support that—perimenopause is also the dawn of a new phase of life. Try embracing the change that's in the air by exploring a new hobby that will teach you new things, expose you to new people, and usher in new experiences—whether that's pickleball, gardening, playing guitar, learning a language, or something else. This tip is also about making space for play in your life, and allowing yourself to be a beginner.

Track your symptoms. With so many varied symptoms, it can be hard to know where to start. Doing some journaling about what you're experiencing and how you're feeling might help you determine what's bothering you the most.

Check your self-talk. It's easy to think or say things like "I look like hell" when you see yourself in the mirror, "I'm falling apart" when another symptom crops up, or "I never want to have sex again" when your libido has gone missing. Try telling yourself the kinds of things you'd say to a friend who shared that she felt unrecognizable to herself, whether that's something like "You look great," "Your body is going through a beneficial reorganization," or "You will come out of this." A little mindset shift can go a long way toward making this transitional period less stressful. As I've mentioned several times in this book, I find cognitive behavioral therapy very impactful for rewriting unhelpful thoughts.

Give yourself some space. Think about what things you can say no to or delegate to give yourself some time and energy to focus on yourself.

Eat more legumes and vegetables. A plant-based diet rich in soy has been shown to reduce vasomotor symptoms.[4] Soy and beans are also rich in protein and fiber—the two categories of food you'll hear me talk about a lot in chapters 8 and 9.

Take a targeted approach to your outlier symptoms. See chapter 10, "Targeted Treatments for Solo Symptoms," for guidance on how to mitigate issues like changing body odor, thinning or otherwise shifting hair, and more. While I recommend starting with treatments that have the potential to target multiple symptoms at once, such as HT, sometimes it pays to be hyper-focused on something that's eating away at your quality of life or self-confidence (or both).

HOT FLASHES GOT YOU BAD?

I've talked about hot flashes and their treatments throughout the book, but here's an easy-access compilation of my best advice for surviving this symptom.

Medical Treatments

Estradiol, at the right dose. It is possible to be taking estradiol and still be getting hot flashes. If that's the case, you may need a higher dose. But if you're also experiencing heavy bleeding, work with your clinician (and refer back to chapter 4) to resolve that first, as taking estrogen can increase bleeding if you are still menstruating.

Progesterone. Low progesterone can sometimes contribute to hot flashes. While taking progesterone is not as effective at treating hot flashes as taking estrogen, it can be helpful.

Veozah. This is a nonhormonal, once-daily, FDA-approved medication for treating hot flashes. If you are experiencing heavy bleeding *and* hot flashes, Veozah can be a very helpful alternative to taking estrogen, which can increase bleeding. I also have some patients who take both Veozah and estrogen to stop the hot flashes.

Brisdelle (paroxetine salt). This antidepressant, technically a selective serotonin reuptake inhibitor (SSRI), also has FDA approval to treat hot flashes.

Combined oral contraceptives, which means birth control that contains both a synthetic progesterone (such as norethindrone or drospirenone) and estrogen (in the form of ethinyl estradiol). This type of birth control can both stop ovulation, thanks to the progesterone component; and reduce symptoms of lowering estrogen.

Things You Can Do on Your Own

Avoid common triggers. While these things may *not* kick off hot flashes for you—meaning, you don't necessarily have to give all of these things up—some women do. Common hot flash triggers include alcohol (yet another reason to drink less!), caffeine, spicy food, and hot beverages. You could also have a different trigger altogether. Try to approach your hot flashes with a spirit of research and investigation—perhaps something is playing a causative role, which you could avoid or minimize.

Adapt to your environment. Hot flashes happen because the hypothalamus has a hard time regulating your internal temperature when the temperature in your external environment changes. It's like estrogen is the dial on your internal thermostat and when it declines, your temperature goes a little haywire. While no one has absolute control over their external environment, you can do what you can to adapt to yours.

This means dressing in layers so that if the temperature in your space rises, you can remove layers to feel cooler. You can also carry a personal fan—I like the ones you can wear around your neck—and embrace the large water bottle trend and keep one filled with cool water with you at all times. (Drinking the water can help, as can pouring a little bit on your wrists.) It also means keeping your bedroom cool—sixty-five degrees tends to be a good temperature for promoting sleep. There are also mattress toppers, sheets, pillows, and pajamas all designed to help you stay cool at night.

Breathe it out. Just like slow, deep breaths can help calm your nervous system in any stressful situation (a fight with your partner, a traffic jam, giving birth), deep breathing can also help steady you during a hot flash, and it may even lessen the intensity or shorten the duration.

Consider cognitive behavioral therapy (CBT). There is a psychological aspect to hot flashes, and CBT can help you reduce the perceived intensity and keep your stress levels a little lower while you are experiencing them. CBT has also been shown to help manage insomnia and modify behaviors that might be contributing to your hot flashes, such as drinking alcohol.

Try self-hypnosis. The Menopause Society endorses this evidence-based form of relaxation for managing hot flashes and night sweats, as well as the insomnia they can bring with them. The Evia app (eviamenopause.com) guides you through research-backed self-hypnotherapy techniques—all you have to do is press play and follow along.

Experiment with supplements and herbs that have a track record of helping some women mitigate hot flashes, including Equelle, ashwagandha, black cohosh, or Estroven. Just keep your clinician apprised of what you're taking so they can monitor for any potential medicine interactions.

Why Your Libido May Be Tanking

If I had a dollar for every patient who has confessed to me that her interest in sex is either dwindling or nonexistent, I'd be able to take my family of five on a very nice vacation. Or two. So, trust me when I say that you are not alone. There are many reasons why you might not be interested in sex right now, some that are physical, and many that are more psychological or even logistical. Let's start with the physical first.

As we've learned, sex can become painful due to dipping estrogen, and libido can lessen as a result of declining testosterone. If you're experiencing pain during sex, I suggest treating that first, as even if your libido rebounds, you still won't feel like having sex if it hurts.

As we've covered, lowering estrogen levels have a direct impact on the moisture, strength, and pH balance of the vaginal tissue. The changes perimenopause can usher in for your vagina (as well as your vulva and clitoris) can result in sex not feeling good anymore, whether that's a lessening of sensitivity or outright pain. Painful intercourse breeds more painful intercourse because your brain starts to anticipate that pain is coming, which then blocks arousal and tightens your muscles (a medical condition called vaginismus), all of which makes sex worse.

Along with the lack of moisture and the weakening of the tissues that declining estrogen can cause, it can also reduce blood flow, and without blood flow, you experience reduced arousal as well as lessened sensitivity, which can mean trouble reaching climax. So maybe sex doesn't outright hurt, but it's less pleasurable and more frustrating for you and your partner, which can result in less of a drive to do it.

Testosterone may be declining now, too, and that can bring libido down with it.

Remember, testosterone is just as much a female hormone as it is a male hormone. It plays an important role in many facets of women's sexual health, including desire, arousal, and orgasm. In addition, some clinical trials show that supplementing with testosterone can improve cognitive performance and musculoskeletal health in postmenopausal women.[5]

Testosterone doesn't decline as reliably as estrogen and progesterone do—for this reason, I recommend getting your levels checked before contemplating whether to add it to your treatment plan. While many women will experience declining levels as they age, testosterone doesn't always fall with the advent of perimenopause and menopause—some women have testosterone that stays in a normal range of 4 to 50 ng/dL their whole lives. (In comparison, the normal range of testosterone for men is between 200 and 500 ng/dL.)

And sometimes, the symptoms of perimenopause just don't make you feel very sexy. If you're exhausted, if your body is changing, if you have lost self-confidence because you don't recognize yourself in the mirror, you're probably not going to feel as interested in getting it on.

Taking a big-picture perspective, the ultimate purpose of the sex drive is reproduction. As you near menopause and your reproductive window gets smaller, I believe your reptilian brain knows that there isn't the same need for sex, and sex moves lower on the list of physiological priorities. So many patients tell me they would rather snuggle, talk, or sleep than have sex; honestly, I can relate.

Especially if you've had children, it's almost like the body is saying, "We can move on now." But it does not have to stay like this forever, and hormone therapy is often helpful. It's also necessary to note that this is just one aspect of declining libido, and it does carry an assumption that you're in a heterosexual relationship and may not apply to women in same-sex relationships or women who are single by choice.

Sex moves up on the list of things to devote time and energy to when you're not exhausted, feeling stressed, and you're no longer worried about everyone else. It's hard to prioritize sex without tending to your four pillars of health (which I cover in chapter 9, "The Silent Symptoms"—don't skip that chapter!) so that you are rested, your mood is in a good place, and you're feeling good about your body.

Many women come into my office and say, "I don't want to have sex and I need to fix this ASAP!" But it's not as simple as just giving you estrogen or testosterone. While it is an exciting fact that there are now medications for women's libido (which I'll cover in this chapter), they're not exactly the female equivalent of Viagra. Viagra affects the penis and the penis only, while medications for women's libido affect the brain because our brains play a huge role in our sex life.

Importantly, there is a lot more to sexual health than hormones and physiology. Your environment, life circumstances, mental health, and relationship also play a huge role. If you're caring for an aging or ill parent, if you're worried about your child's mental health, or if you have financial troubles or are stressed about the state of the world—or any combination of these factors—it can have a direct impact on your sex life and your libido.

By the time you're in your forties, you may have been with your partner for several years. That shared history, both good and bad, can affect your bond. Novelty inevitably wears off, which can lower sexual attraction and the intense drive you may have once had to get your hands on each other. It can feel like there's not a lot of mystery left. Maybe you have trust issues. Or maybe you've fallen into a rut where doing the same things no longer has an enjoyable result.

Living with children can also do a number on libido. Right now, my house feels like the unsexiest place possible. There are toys in my bed, little piles of sports equipment and backpacks and shoes everywhere, and all the clutter reads to me like a giant, never-ending to-do list. Not very alluring.

These are all pieces of what's known as the biopsychosocial foundations of sexual health, which is a fancy way of noting that there are many different factors influencing your sexual wellness beyond tissues and hormones. In my practice we use the Female Sexual Function Index (FSFI)—a self-reported questionnaire that assesses six areas of sexual function, including arousal, desire, lubrication, orgasm, pain, and satisfaction. I often hear patients say, "I didn't realize how bad things were until I filled out this questionnaire," because it's easy to dismiss the signs that your sex life could use some help, as the changes can creep up slowly and there are simply so many other things vying for your attention. (I've included a link to the FSFI at heatherhirschmd.com so you can get a clearer picture of your relationship to your sex life.) I recommend filling out the questionnaire because it might shed more light on your experience throughout the perimenopausal journey.

Before we discuss treatment options for low libido, take a minute to honestly assess how important improving your sex life is at this particular moment. Determining the best treatment plan for you really depends on your full suite of symptoms, priorities, medical history, and sense of urgency that influence which part of hormone therapy to start with. For that reason, whenever a patient tells me, "I'd like my sex to get better," I always ask, "For you, or for your partner, or both?" If the answer is "For my partner," I suggest moving libido down the priority list, because nothing we do will be significantly effective if we're doing it for someone else. I'd rather see you prioritize sleep or address brain fog, because those will make *you* feel better—and when you do, you may genuinely feel more interested in tending to your sex life.

MEDICATIONS THAT CAN LOWER LIBIDO

If you're taking any of these medications, share with your doctor that you are experiencing low libido and discuss any possible alternatives or different dosing that might be appropriate. Please do not stop any medication cold turkey without consulting with your doctor first.

ADHD medications: amphetamines (Adzenys ER, Adzenys XR-ODT, Dyanavel XR); or dextroamphetamines/amphetamines (Adderall, Adderall XR, Mydayis)

Antianxiety drugs: alprazolam (Xanax); diazepam (Valium)

Antidepressants: duloxetine (Cymbalta); paroxetine (Paxil); sertraline (Zoloft); venlafaxine (Effexor)

Antifungals: ketoconazole (Nizoral)

Antihistamines: diphenhdyramine (Benadryl); or chlorpheniramine (Chlor-Trimeton)

Antiseizure medications: carbamazepine (Tegretol)
Beta-blockers: propranolol (Inderal LA, InnoPran XL); or metoprolol (Kapspargo Sprinkle, Lopressor, Toprol-XL)
Birth control pills: (as all birth control pills lower testosterone)
Cancer treatments: such as chemotherapy and radiation
Diuretics: chlorthalidone; hydrochlorothiazide (Microzide)
Heartburn drugs: famotidine (Pepcid)
Heart failure medications: digoxin (Lanoxin); spironolactone (Aldactone)
Hypertension drugs: atenolol (Tenormin); clonidine (Catapres); metoprolol (Lopressor); methyldopa (Aldomet)

Treatments That Can Help Libido (in the Order I Typically Recommend Them)

If low libido is part of your symptom set, I would measure your testosterone levels to help determine if they are low and, if so, supplementing testosterone might make sense. I'd also review the medications you're taking, as some can negatively impact sexual desire.

Topical Vaginal Estrogen

If sex is painful, there is no better way to restore the health of your tissues than to start using topical vaginal estrogen. Actually, let me restate that. If sex is painful, you *need* vaginal estrogen, as it is the only way to truly reverse the changes resulting from the genitourinary syndrome of menopause.

There are many good reasons to use vaginal estrogen—more moisture, a better pH balance, stronger tissues, and less risk of urinary infections among them. One benefit I don't think we talk about enough is that restoring the health of the tissue can also open the door to more pleasure, which also means more stress relief and more bonding (as orgasm triggers the release of the love hormone oxytocin).

The fact is, nothing else will reverse the atrophy of the tissue except for estrogen, whether it is administered locally or systemically (and some women will need both—yes, that is common!). While lube can be your best friend in perimenopause and beyond, it really only prevents chafing from the friction of intercourse. Vaginal moisturizers can help lock in water so there's more of a barrier. But neither does anything to remedy the atrophying of your tissue or to restore the acidic pH except estrogen.

Taking systemic estrogen can absolutely help, too, but approximately 40 percent of women taking HT also need and use local vaginal estrogen. Remember, the highest concentration of estrogen receptors is in the lower genitourinary tract—this very sensitive part of the body can sometimes just use a little more support. It is normal and safe to use both systemic and local estrogen *if* your symptoms warrant it. I hear from women that doctors are guiding them away from using both because they think it's unnecessary or dangerous, and that's not true.

Because vaginal estrogen is local, no significant amount enters the bloodstream and travels throughout the body, which makes it safe for all women, even cancer survivors. In fact, a study that followed women using vaginal estrogen for eighteen years found that they had no increased risk of cardiovascular disease or cancer compared to women who did not use it.[6]

Testosterone

There is widespread agreement among medical professionals and associations that testosterone is helpful for treating low libido in women, as stated in the 2019 global consensus position statement on testosterone.[7] Despite this unity in medical opinion, maddeningly, there is no FDA-approved formulation of testosterone for female dosing currently on the market.

Although there isn't consensus on testosterone's other potential benefits for women (which I'm not terribly surprised about), in my clinical experience, women report that testosterone has helped them with mood, joint aches and pains, muscle mass (which can also help protect against a declining bone density), and sleep.

Because there is no testosterone prescription medication formulated for female dosing, what most perimenopause-savvy clinicians recommend is using the male version of testosterone—which comes in a transdermal gel (called Testim or AndroGel)—but only using one-tenth of the dose suggested for men. These often come preportioned in a packet or a tube, so I tell patients to make one packet or tube last about ten days.

Some clinicians may prescribe a compounded testosterone gel or cream, which can be helpful because the compounding pharmacy can tailor the daily amount to be a bit more consistent, which is something to discuss with your clinician. I typically don't recommend compounding hormones, but in this case, since there is no FDA equivalent that comes prepackaged for the female, it's another option to consider.

There's one form of testosterone therapy I advise against: pellets. These are injected under your skin and contain a high level of systemic testosterone that is designed to last for three months. These are not covered by insurance and hence are typically very costly, and once they're in, they are not easily removed. If your clinician recommends pellets, especially without any mention of the FDA-approved HT formulations that exist (albeit for men), find another clinician.

I consider adding testosterone only after we have taken an inventory of any biopsychosocial aspects (such as stress levels and relationship dynamics) and have tended to the four pillars of health (including diet, movement, sleep, and mental health). If those things are in a pretty good place and your desire is still low, it's a good opportunity to consider adding testosterone.

Systemic Estrogen

While not a direct treatment for low libido, systemic estrogen can help make sex better by supporting the tissues of the vagina, vulva, and clitoris, thus increasing blood flow, which helps with arousal and sensitivity. Refer back to the sidebar "Treatments That Can Help with Hot Flashes and Brain Fog" earlier in this chapter for more information on using systemic estrogen as part of your treatment plan.

Prescription Medications for Low Libido

As I've covered elsewhere, Addyi is a nonhormonal medication that is FDA-approved for treating low libido. The once-daily oral medication is a dopamine agonist, meaning it works in the brain to activate your reward-and-pleasure circuitry. Patients who have tried it tell me it also helps them with mood and sleep, which is a nice side benefit.

Vyleesi is a short-acting injection that also works in the brain to increase activity in your reward-and-pleasure circuits. Because you use it only when you want to have sex, it's a nice option if you don't want to take a medication every day, add to your pill burden, or open the door to interactions with other medications you may be taking (although there are no interactions with HT). Vyleesi works best when you use it sparingly, so it might be something to consider if libido is more important for your relationship than it is for you personally, for example.

While I generally recommend testosterone for low libido first, if there's some reason you don't want to take testosterone—maybe you're leery of a potential side effect such as unwanted facial hair or acne, or your testosterone levels are actually in a good place (it may even be elevated if you are chronically stressed), these medications can be a great alternative.

Things You Can Do on Your Own for Sexual Health

Prioritize novelty. In terms of strengthening the connection between you and your partner, appealing to your brain can help here, too. We tend to think of neuroplasticity—the process of forging new connections between neurons in your brain by learning new things—as an important part of cognition that can protect brain health, but it can help your relationships, too. How can you do new things together as a couple? It could be a sport (I recently learned how to ski, or tried, anyway, so that my husband and I can have a new way to connect especially during the winter months when it can get awfully gray where we live in upstate

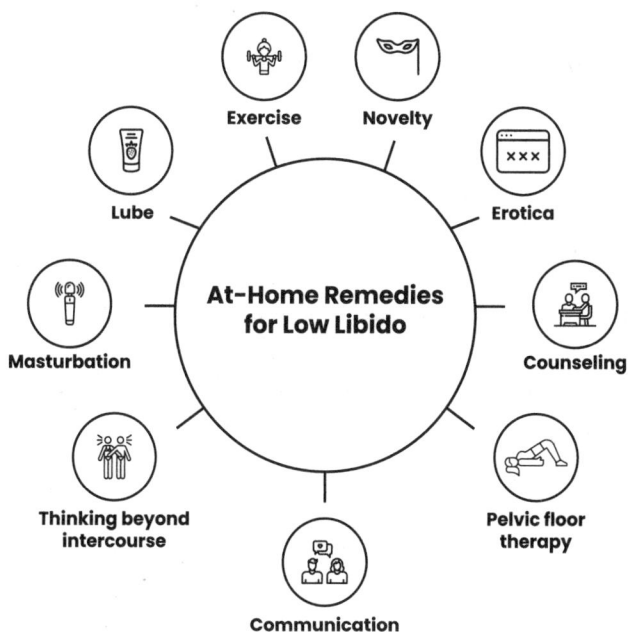

Exercise · Novelty · Erotica · Counseling · Pelvic floor therapy · Communication · Thinking beyond intercourse · Masturbation · Lube

At-Home Remedies for Low Libido

New York), traveling someplace you haven't been before, taking a class together, or simply seeking out new-to-you things to do in your community, like checking out restaurants you've never been to or visiting the tourist attractions you've always driven right past.

Spark your desire. The desire for sex can become more responsive as you get into your forties and beyond, meaning, it's less likely to arise all on its own and may need someone or something to kick it off. To get started, I recommend Rosy, a doctor-created app that, in addition to offering sexual wellness education and access to a community of women who are prioritizing their sexual health, also has a large library of free, woman-focused erotic content, including romantic and erotic short stories to help get you in the mood.

Embrace lube. To be clear, the best way for restoring vaginal moisture (among many other genitourinary benefits) is localized vaginal estrogen. However, whether you use vaginal estrogen or you don't, lube is still a reliable, safe, and convenient way to promote slip and slide. And science has shown that women are more likely to experience orgasm when they use lube.[8] (Really, need I say more?) Just make sure your lube is water-based if you're using condoms, as silicone-based lubes can cause a condom to break.

Tend to your pelvic floor. While not technically related to hormonal decline, it is possible for the muscles of your pelvic floor to contribute to painful sex because they can get tight, especially if you sit a lot or have had children, and too many Kegels can make an already tight pelvic floor even worse. Many of my patients have found pelvic floor physical therapy extremely helpful. There's also the Milli, a device designed to help relax tight pelvic floor muscles, increase blood flow, and reduce pain. Learn more at hellomilli.com.

Consider couples counseling. As we've covered, generally speaking, low libido or diminished interest in sex often has mental and emotional roots. You're going through so many changes, and your relationships may be, too. Seeing a therapist together can help you improve your communication skills and better understand each other. It doesn't mean your relationship is in trouble; it simply means you'd like it to be even better. See "Appendix B: Resources" at the back of this book for guidance on where to look for a therapist.

Try self-stimulation. Masturbation (with or without a vibrator, and with or without a partner present) is a great way to explore what feels good to you now and invite a little more pleasure into your life. While you don't necessarily need one, the sex toy industry is booming—there is likely a device out there that hits you in all the right places, and using a vibrator has been shown to help achieve orgasm.[9]

Experiment beyond intercourse. Penetrative sex isn't the be-all and end-all, which is a good thing, because it just may not be feeling all that good at the moment. Play around with mutual masturbation, oral sex, and sensual massage. Your body is changing, so your definition of "having sex" may need to change, too.

Get that blood flowing. Yes, I'm going to recommend exercise... again. But arousal depends on blood flow, and the best way to boost circulation is to get moving. Yoga that opens up your hips and pelvis, squats, rowing, spinning, and cycling can directly stimulate your pelvic region, but any kind of movement is helpful.

Open up the lines of communication. If perimenopause can be confusing to women, imagine how mystifying it can be for their partners. They may not understand that things could be feeling different for you. The brain is such an important part of the sexual response—use yours to open up a dialogue that can help you both feel more connected.

CHAPTER 8

Gaining Weight for No (Apparent) Reason

Naomi had been trim all her life without really trying. Even after she had her two children, her weight returned to baseline within a few months after delivery. But now, at forty-seven, it feels like she's gained eight pounds overnight, even though nothing in her diet or activity level changed. All of the waistbands of her pants are now too tight, and even though she's cut out all sweets and started taking long, brisk walks most mornings, she can't seem to shed the weight.

Kelly always jokingly called herself a Renaissance woman because she had curves that were fashionable in earlier eras. She accepted her body, even though she grew up in the 1990s when heroin chic was all the rage and diet culture was rampant. When she put on weight after having kids, she adapted to her new normal. But once she hit her mid-forties, she felt like the needle on the scale just kept creeping higher and nothing she did seemed to help. Now her doctor is telling her she's prediabetic and she needs to lose weight. But how?

At any time of life, weight gain is complicated. When perimenopause enters the picture, it gets even more so.

If you have a uterus and ovaries, are at midlife, and you have recently gained extra weight that you just can't shed, I have some important things to tell you:

You are likely not imagining it.

You are not alone.

It is not your fault.

It's time to shift our focus away from the number on the scale and toward better barometers of health. The good news is that there are many helpful approaches to countering the metabolic changes that peri- menopause can usher in, and we are going to dive into all of them in this chapter.

In my practice, 75 percent of my patients tell me they've gained weight, a fact that often makes them wonder what they're doing wrong— even though most of them also say that they haven't changed their life- style, the way they're eating, or how much they're moving.

I want to be very clear: We have to stop thinking of weight gain as something that you do to yourself. This goes for everyone at all times of life (for reasons I'll unpack in this chapter), but *especially* for women at midlife. If you came to this book because you've recently gained weight and don't know (a) why; or (b) what to do about it, I'll comment on the (a) part now by telling you it's due to a combination of things that are out- side your control. Your hormonal transition plays a major role, yes, but so does the culture and reality in which we live. In a nutshell: It is really easy to gain weight and really hard to take it off and keep it off. So let's talk about how to navigate this tricky yet important subject.

GAINING WEIGHT FOR NO (APPARENT) REASON SYMPTOMS AT A GLANCE

Hallmarks:

- Increase in waist size
- Weight creeping up
- Increase in abdominal fat
- Losing muscle tone
- Increase in bra size (breasts are fatty tissue!)

Causative Factors:

- Declining estrogen
- Subsequent disruption in insulin function
- Increase in hunger cues
- Decrease in satiety cues
- Living in a culture with an abundance of highly processed foods and fast-food options.

First, let's look at the cultural reasons why weight gain happens. To start, you have to really try to seek out whole, unprocessed foods. According to one estimate published in the journal *Nature Communications*, 73 percent of our food supply is ultra-processed; these foods have been modified from their original form and engineered to be so delicious as to be craveable (or even addictive), while also being stripped of many of their inherent nutrients and "enhanced" by preservatives and other chemical additives to make them more visually attractive and shelf-stable.[1] Ultra-processed foods typically contain tons of carbohydrates with little fiber and are packed with sugar, salt, and fat to make them irresistible. A quick way to determine if something is ultra-processed is to look at the ingredient list. (Or see if my kids like it. But I'm joking. Mostly.) If there are words you don't recognize and can't pronounce, you know you're eating things that have been greatly modified away from their original state. Not surprisingly, most fast food, frozen meals, and packaged foods fit the ultra-processed bill.

There has been a lot of research out of Brazil looking at the health impacts of eating a lot of ultra-processed foods, and the findings are disturbing. While some of their findings may feel obvious—that a diet high in ultra-processed foods is linked to weight gain and an increase in waist size,[2] even more upsettingly, they have also found that a diet high in ultra-processed foods is responsible for 22 percent of premature deaths from cardiovascular disease and a third of premature deaths from all causes.[3]

But who can blame anyone for reaching for ultra-processed foods when they are incredibly convenient? So many of us, especially peri-menopausal women in the thick of career or caregiving or both, are living a hyper-fast-paced lifestyle that certainly doesn't leave a lot of time for food shopping, cooking, and cleaning up. Ultra-processed foods are everywhere—even the checkout aisle at stores like Old Navy and Home Depot are lined with candy, bags of chips, and cold soda ready to grab and go. Plus, these foods are shelf-stable and taste the same every time—with the exception of the continual variations, like green Oreos for St. Patrick's Day and Extra-Toasty Cheez-Its, so that we get pulled back in by the novelty if we get tired of the same old flavor experience. I want to be clear that I am no exception—I frequently get my daughter Wendy's on the way to lacrosse practice because it's easier than packing something, and I know she'll eat it. My most regular snack these days is the Trader Joe's animal crackers my toddler loves. My family gets takeout more times than I'd like to admit. Yes, meal planning and prepping help, but I can manage that for about two weeks at most before I get derailed.

It's not just that nutrient-poor convenience foods are everywhere in the real world—we're also constantly being exposed to marketing that promotes them. That means they're taking up rent-free space in our minds as well as on store shelves. According to the University of Connecticut Rudd Center for Food Policy and Health, food makers, beverage companies, and restaurants spend $14 billion a year on marketing their products. More than 80 percent of these dollars go to promoting fast food, sweets, and unhealthy snacks. Compare that to the $1 billion budget that the US Centers for Disease Control and Prevention (CDC) has available to spend on promoting healthy eating and disease prevention, and you can see the cards are stacked in favor of the unhealthy stuff.[4]

Portion sizes have also crept up—according to the CDC, a small order of fries in the 1980s was just over two ounces and contained 210 calories. Today, the average order of fries is about six ounces and contains 610 calories—or about three times more fries and more calories. Even our dishes and glasses are bigger than they used to be. As an example, the plates I received as wedding gifts from Pottery Barn don't fit in the cabinets in my house that was built in 1992!

We've become accustomed to eating greater amounts of food—particularly in the forms of sugar and refined carbs—with fewer nutrients, especially fiber, which slows the release of sugar into the bloodstream; and protein, which helps us build muscle and feel full. As a result, our blood sugar spikes, which means that we also have too much insulin—a hormone that moves blood sugar out of the bloodstream and into the cells. High insulin kicks off a hormonal cascade that prioritizes storing extra glucose as fat, and also promotes strong carbohydrate cravings to replenish the glucose. This is why people who start taking insulin to treat their diabetes can often gain weight, even though their blood sugar is under better control. Insulin also brings blood sugar down, which sounds like a good thing, except that when those glucose levels drop precipitously (like after a sugary donut), the body sends hunger cues in an effort to get more carbs to stabilize blood sugar levels again.

On top of all this, we live in a fat-phobic society, where bigger bodies—especially female bodies, and even more the bodies of Black or brown women, who often face discrimination based on their race as well as their size—are harshly judged. It's too easy for women to internalize the message that smaller is better, so when perimenopausal weight gain happens, it can trigger all kinds of worries and unkind self-talk. And the stress of being exposed to such judgment also takes its own toll on our health.

Phew, it's a lot! And that's even before we factor in perimenopause.

The Link Between Perimenopause and Weight Gain

While the medical research community isn't in 100 percent agreement on exactly how female reproductive hormonal transition at midlife contributes to weight gain, we do know from large-scale studies such as the Women's Health Initiative and reviews that analyzed data from multiple studies that women who take hormone therapy have lower rates of type 2 diabetes compared to women who do not take hormone therapy.[5] This suggests a positive link between estrogen and improved insulin function (or insulin sensitivity, as we say in medical lingo).

Remember, the more estrogen declines, the more insulin resistance and insulin levels tend to rise. The higher your insulin level is, the more your cells get the cue to store excess glucose as fat instead of converting it to glycogen and using it for fuel. That's why weight gain is a common symptom of perimenopause—and why shedding that weight isn't as simple as eating less and moving more, because without estrogen, your insulin will still be out of whack.

There are other aspects of perimenopause that contribute to weight gain:

- The sleep disruptions that tend to happen during perimenopause kick off their own hormonal cascade that increases both appetite and fat storage. A lack of sufficient sleep may also lower your metabolism, as well as make you more lethargic the next day—and less likely to engage in movement. The fatigue that often settles in during perimenopause can also make you crave quick-burning carbs for energy. (Craving Twizzlers at 2:00 p.m. to get through the last meeting? Yup, that's the result of a lack of solid sleep.)

- Perimenopause can do a number on your mood, as we've covered, and that could cause you to crave comfort food to ease anxiety or boost mood or energy if you're dealing with depression. Depression also makes you unmotivated to exercise and less likely to want to cook nutritious food.

- Perimenopause tends to start at the busiest time in a woman's life, which may mean you're not exercising because you feel like there just isn't time for it in your schedule. And, if you have children, chances are they're past the toddler years, when you were constantly running after them.

- Declining testosterone levels can cause you to lose muscle mass. And since muscle has a higher metabolic rate (meaning, it burns more calories just to maintain itself than fat or bone), when it declines your metabolism can lower, too, making it that much easier to gain weight without changing anything about your daily routine.

While the precise chemical process that causes weight gain in perimenopause hasn't been pinpointed by science (yet), it's my professional opinion that the underlying physiological reason why women experience these shifts in weight at midlife is that we are experiencing a fundamental hormonal disruption. I think of the relationship between perimenopause and weight gain as two sets of interlocking gears. The first gear is the reproductive hormones—your estrogen, progesterone, and testosterone—which then turns the second gear, which is your metabolic hormones, including insulin, ghrelin, and leptin. As the first gear slows down, the second gear gets out of balance as well. Double whammy.

How many calories you eat or how much you exercise isn't going to impact your reproductive hormone gear. A classic example of how these two gears make weight loss more complicated for women is when a husband and wife decide to go on a diet. The husband stops drinking beer and soda and loses twenty pounds, while the wife cleans up her entire diet and starts working out several times a week and barely loses three pounds. Why? Because the wife's reproductive hormone gear is not functioning well and it's blocking her access to her second gear, while the husband's efforts directly influence the function of his metabolic hormone gear.

Weight Matters—but Not as Much as We've Been Taught to Think

Doctors are not immune to fat phobia, which can cause them to blame weight gain for a lot of health issues that have other root causes—like, for example, the fatigue and increase in cholesterol many women experience in their forties that are actually caused by declining sex hormones (we'll talk more about the cholesterol piece in chapter 9).

We know that obesity (defined as a BMI of 31 or higher) is linked to higher rates of diabetes, heart disease, and cancer. But there is research that suggests being overweight (defined as having a BMI of between 25 and 30) isn't in itself as much of a health issue as we have been taught that it is, especially when looking at weight's impact on lifespan. A large review of multiple studies published in the *Journal of the American Medical Association* found that being overweight was associated with significantly *less* risk of dying than being a "normal" weight (although, as our food supply has changed and we've grown heavier in general, what is even normal?). Moreso, even having a BMI of 31–35 (technically referred to as stage 1 obesity in the research) carried the same risk of mortality as being a "normal" weight.[6] Other research out of Denmark has found that people with the lowest risk of dying have a BMI of 27, firmly in the "overweight" category.[7] And a 2024 review of twenty studies found that being physically active and fit was a stronger predictor of longevity than weight—even someone who technically has obesity is about half as likely to die as someone with a normal weight but a low fitness level.[8]

All that being said, there are a couple of troubling health risks that perimenopausal weight gain can bring with it. The first is that belly fat, which is where perimenopausal weight gain typically settles, poses extra risks to our health because it is linked to an increased risk of metabolic syndrome, a precursor to heart disease (which I outline in chapter 9). And I have said it before, but it's such an easily overlooked fact that I will say it again—heart disease is the number one killer of women.

Another valid health risk of gaining weight is an increased likelihood of developing sleep apnea, where your airways close periodically while you are sleeping, cutting off the oxygen supply to your brain and causing you to wake up multiple times throughout the night (even if you don't remember it happening). Sleep apnea is linked to an increased risk of high blood pressure, heart disease, type 2 diabetes, and memory loss. (There's more on sleep apnea in chapter 9, which is about the silent symptoms of perimenopause that all women are at risk of developing.)

And thanks to our cultural attitudes about body size, gaining weight for no apparent reason can lead to a pretty potent stew of worry and other negative feelings, which can then start impacting your mental health and your confidence. Believe me, I understand the desire to fit into your clothes and feel confident in your body.

So you don't want to completely ignore weight gain, but you don't want to put too much stock into what the scale says, either. It's a delicate balance that we will walk through in this chapter.

One truth is this: It is absolutely vital that you eat a healthy diet and get plenty of movement (in fact, diet and exercise are two of the four pillars of health that I cover in chapter 9). Another, countervailing truth, is that it's time to shift focus away from the numbers on the scale as a barometer of how healthy we are. After all, we don't have a ton of control over what those numbers are, for all the reasons we've covered thus far.

Instead, the numbers you want to pay attention to are the metrics listed in the "Metabolic Syndrome and Perimenopause" sidebar in chapter 1. Briefly, you want to aim for a waist size of thirty-five inches or lower and keep an eye on your cholesterol, triglycerides, LDL cholesterol, hemoglobin A1C (a measure of your average glucose levels over the last three months to assess for prediabetes or diabetes), and blood pressure. Adopting the foundational diet and movement strategies I outline in the "What You Can Do on Your Own" section of this chapter will help you keep these numbers in a good range. Just as importantly, you can rest assured that you're taking good care of yourself and can then focus your attention and energy on accepting and loving your body even if it has changed.

There are also medications—some new, some tried-and-true—that can either help address the underlying endocrine disruption that is likely contributing to your weight gain (if you guessed hormone therapy, ding, ding, ding—you're right!—although other meds can help regulate insulin and blood sugar) or help reduce your appetite and help you lose a significant amount of weight (if you have a significant amount of weight to lose), such as semaglutides (e.g., Wegovy and Ozempic). Although these meds are generally well-tolerated, safe, and effective, they aren't for everyone. We'll cover how to choose which, if any, are right for you in the next section.

MEDICATIONS THAT CAN CAUSE WEIGHT GAIN

If you're taking any of these meds, talk to your doctor about their possible side effects first and share your concerns about weight gain—perhaps you can take a lower dose or explore alternatives. Please do not come off any medication cold turkey without consulting with your doctor first.

Anticonvulsants: carbamazepine (Tegretol, Equetro); gabapentin (Gralise, Neurontin); pregabalin (Lyrica); valproate (Depakene, Depakote); vigabatrin (Sabril)

Antidepressants: amitriptyline (Elavil); citalopram (Celexa); doxepin (Silenor); escitalopram (Lexapro); nortriptyline (Pamelor); paroxetine (Paxil); phenelzine (Nardil); sertraline (Zoloft)

Antihistamines (over-the-counter): cyproheptadine (Periactin); cetirizine (Zyrtec); desloratadine (Clarinex); diphenhydramine (Benadryl); fexofenadine (Allegra); hydroxyzine (Vistaril)

Antipsychotics: clozapine (Clozaril); olanzapine (Zyprexa); quetiapine (Seroquel); risperidone (Risperdal)

Beta-blockers: acebutolol (Sectral); atenolol (Tenormin); bisoprolol (Zebeta); metoprolol (Lopressor, Toprol-XL); nadolol (Corgard); nebivolol (Bystolic); propranolol (Inderal LA, InnoPran XL)

Birth control shot: medroxyprogesterone acetate (Depo-Provera)

Diabetes meds: insulin and sulfonylureas, such as gliclazide (Diamicron); glibenclamide (Glynase); glipizide; glimepiride; glyburide

Migraine meds: divalproex sodium (Depakote); propranolol (Inderal)

Steroids: cortisone (Cortone); hydrocortisone (Cortef, Hydrocortone); methylprednisolone (Medrol); prednisone (Deltasone, Predone, Sterapred)

Treatments That Can Help with Weight Loss (in the Order I Typically Recommend Them)

For patients who tell me that they are gaining weight and don't know why, the labs I recommend are the following: thyroid panel; a complete metabolic panel (to see how well the liver is functioning); HbA1C; and a lipid panel to assess cholesterol levels to determine if the patient has metabolic syndrome, as this may influence our treatment plan (if metabolic syndrome, prediabetes, or diabetes is present, weight-loss medications may be a fit).

Additionally, I'll ask what prescriptions they are currently taking as certain medications can cause weight gain—see the "Medications That Can Cause Weight Gain" sidebar to check if something you're taking might be playing a role. And I'll ask about their sleep habits, as we know that sleep is easily disrupted in perimenopause and it plays an important role in your appetite, energy levels, and metabolism, and also your current diet and exercise regimen.

Once we have these results in hand, and can rule out things like thyroid hormone dysfunction, we'll talk through a full spectrum of options for addressing weight gain, including the foundational nutrition and movement strategies that every perimenopausal woman needs to adopt in order to lay a foundation of generational health that will help carry her into and through the second half of life.

Here are the medical treatment options that may be helpful in supporting metabolic health.

Hormone Therapy

Because the vast majority of perimenopausal weight gain has an endocrine disruption at its root, my first recommendation to the vast majority of my patients is to consider hormone therapy, especially if they are symptomatic. Often, I will recommend that my patients start with either estradiol or progesterone and estradiol if they are experiencing sleep disruptions. While not a treatment for weight loss per se—and to be clear,

HT is not FDA-approved for weight loss—we know that hormone therapy can improve insulin sensitivity, and that can help ward off additional weight gain and remove one of the obstacles to losing weight, especially if following the diet and lifestyle recommendations in "Things You Can Do on Your Own."

My patients report that going on hormone therapy helps them feel like their metabolism is "running again" and that it's helping them sleep better, which makes it easier not to overeat carbs and to have the energy for some form of exercise they enjoy.

This is what happened to my patient Jenny, who was in late perimenopause when she came to see me. Despite having a very active job and eating plenty of healthy foods like fruits and vegetables—she and her family owned an apple farm—Jenny was gaining weight and her doctor told her that her elevated A1C levels meant she was prediabetic. Over the course of the previous two years, she'd gained fifteen pounds. In addition, she wasn't sleeping well, she was feeling anxious or irritable regularly, sex was no longer feeling good, and her blood pressure had crept up.

Together we decided that Jenny would take progesterone at bedtime to help her sleep and ease her anxiety. Once she was feeling better rested, we added low-dose estrogen for her vaginal dryness and to help her mood—and her insulin—be in a better place. Over the next six months, Jenny had lost the weight she'd gained, her blood pressure went down, and she was enjoying sex again. Her A1C lowered enough to get her out of the prediabetic range. The last time I checked in with her, she hadn't had a period in over a year and was sailing into menopause without a worry!

Wellbutrin

This antidepressant is a dopamine agonist that works by increasing levels of dopamine and norepinephrine in the brain. As such, in addition to producing an uptick in mood, it can increase the activity of the reward circuitry in the brain, reducing the urge to stress eat and also help curb binge eating. Wellbutrin has been shown to help with losing an average of five to seven pounds.[9] Because it is also a mild stimulant, it can help with difficulty concentrating. For these reasons, when I see a woman who reports irritability, brain fog or attention deficit, and a little bit of weight gain (which could be so many of us on any given day, including me), we'll often discuss Wellbutrin as an option *after* we've stabilized her hormone therapy dosage (if HT is appropriate for her), and if she's still dealing with symptoms such as mood disruptions and weight gain.

Pros: Wellbutrin is well-covered by insurance and, therefore, typically inexpensive (about $10 for a thirty-day supply). It doesn't require weaning—if it doesn't work or you don't like the way it feels, you can simply stop taking it.

Cons: Because it's a mild stimulant, Wellbutrin is not a great choice for someone who experiences regular anxiety. In rare cases, it can cause tinnitus (a ringing sound in your ear) that doesn't resolve after you stop taking it. Wellbutrin can also worsen hot flashes, so if you are already experiencing hot flashes regularly, Wellbutrin may not be the best fit.

Metformin

This diabetes drug can be used off-label to lose a little bit of weight—about five to seven pounds, on average. Metformin works primarily by lowering blood sugar levels and helping the body to maintain a steady insulin level, which improves insulin resistance and helps you avoid blood sugar spikes and crashes that can lead to cravings. It also helps you feel fuller longer, and has been shown to support a healthy microbiome, which is likely why it also improves a slow gut transit (i.e., helps to relieve constipation).

It has a reputation of promoting longevity, but that benefit has been noted primarily in animals, and animal studies don't always extend to humans. Science isn't clear on metformin's longevity benefits for nondiabetics, but if your A1C levels are veering into prediabetic territory (which starts at 5.7) or you have type 2 diabetes, metformin can be helpful for more than just a little weight loss.

Pros: As metformin has been around awhile, it is well-studied, considered safe, and is generally well-tolerated.

Cons: Some of its potential side effects are diarrhea and nausea.

Semaglutide Medications (Mounjaro, Ozempic, and Wegovy)
These medications were initially made to help treat diabetes and are also designed for weight loss, and they tend to be very effective. They work by mimicking glucagon-like peptide-1 (GLP-1), a hormone that's produced in the gut and works in the brain to regulate appetite, food intake, and fullness. By binding to the GLP-1 receptors in the brain, semaglutides:

- Decrease appetite by reducing hunger cues from the hormone ghrelin and essentially telling the body you are full.
- Slow the movement of food through the stomach, meaning you feel fuller for longer and increasing the satiety hormone leptin—in fact, some people taking semaglutides will lose their appetite to the point that they forget to eat.
- Increase insulin production in response to an elevation in blood sugar levels, which helps reduce overall insulin resistance (when insulin receptors lose their sensitivity because insulin remains elevated regardless of blood sugar levels, it essentially burns those receptors out)—as well as blood sugar levels.
- Shut off food noise, or thinking about how hungry you are and what you'll eat next, which can relieve a lot of anxiety and free up time and energy for other more productive things. Through this benefit alone, semaglutides can improve mood, although this facet cuts both ways—you can also lose the pleasure and excitement of eating.
- Lower levels of glucagon, a hormone that tells the liver to release glucose into the bloodstream, thereby reducing blood sugar levels—which is particularly helpful for people with type 2 diabetes.
- Promote the burning of calories in general and fat in particular.

Although they may feel like they're new on the scene, the first semaglutide, exenatide (Byetta and Bydureon), was approved for the treatment of type 2 diabetes in 2005. Earlier forms of this class of drugs needed to be injected twice a day, and due to this difficulty of use, the drugs didn't really catch on until they were released in their current form, which requires only a once-a-week injection. Still, because of their long record of use, we know a lot about the long-term safety of these medications.

Semaglutides aren't for losing just a little bit of weight—they are recommended for type 2 diabetics with a body mass index (BMI) of 27 or higher who still have elevated high blood sugars even though they've tried other diabetes medications, or for nondiabetics with a BMI over 30, or for those with a BMI of 27 who also have at least one weight-related condition, such as high blood pressure, high cholesterol, or sleep apnea.

In my clinical experience, women on HT get similar results from using lower doses of semaglutides compared to women who are not on HT. Interesting, huh? This fact only reinforces our hypothesis that estrogen helps regulate insulin.

Pros: These medications are very effective at promoting weight loss and generally well-tolerated. They have been found to have additional health benefits, too, including a reduction in the risks of cardiovascular disease, cardiovascular events such as heart attack or stroke, and death from cardiovascular disease, along with a reduction in HbA1c and, thus, type 2 diabetes. Also, semaglutides are being investigated, with promising preliminary results, for treating polycystic ovarian syndrome, Alzheimer's, Parkinson's, liver disease, and sleep apnea.[10]

Cons: When you stop taking semaglutides, the weight is very likely to come back. That means you need to think of it as a long-term medication, although you can reduce your dosage and interval between injections, as my patient Tabitha did. In her twenties and thirties, Tabitha saw her weight creep up to the point that by her late forties, she was forty pounds heavier, her BMI was 31, and she had developed sleep apnea. Once Tabitha's perimenopause hit full stride, her night sweats and brain fog were leaving her feeling miserable. Because she met the criteria for semaglutides and wanted relief from her sleep apnea, she opted to start Wegovy. Tabitha lost thirty-five pounds and was feeling great, but she noticed that she really missed being able to enjoy certain foods, like the fried seafood and ice cream she and her family savored every summer on their annual trip to Cape Cod. We switched her to a much lower maintenance dosage, with an injection only every two weeks. Later, we decreased the frequency to once every three weeks. Six months later, Tabitha had gained five pounds back, but she was good with that because even though she was eating smaller amounts of her favorite foods than she once did, they didn't make her feel nauseated as had happened when she was on her original dosage.

This is not really a con versus a pro, but more of a reminder: You still need your nutrition and movement to be in a good place.

There are some risks and downsides to semaglutides, including a small increased risk of thyroid cancer (so far seen only in animal studies, but it's something to take into account); and acute kidney injury due to dehydration, gallstones, or pancreatitis. Insurance coverage also varies and the drugs can be quite costly if your insurance doesn't cover them. Some people experience nausea, vomiting, diarrhea, or dehydration on semaglutides. And if you have a history of multiple endocrine neoplasia syndrome type 2 (MEN 2), this is a contradindication.

Appetite-Suppressant Medications

These include Contrave (a combination of bupropion—the generic version of Wellbutrin—and naltrexone, which is used to treat alcohol and opioid addiction and also carries FDA-approval as a weight-loss aid); Adipex (phentermine, a nervous system stimulant); and Qsymia (a combination of phentermine and topiramate—an anticonvulsant), all of which decrease appetite.

Now that semaglutides are available, I recommend appetite-suppressant medications less often, especially as they tend to have a lot of side effects that lower quality of life, including feeling nauseated and out of sorts, but they are a treatment you could discuss with your doctor if semaglutides aren't an option.

Because Contrave contains the opioid blocker naltrexone and can dull the reward circuitry in the brain, it has the potential to short-circuit emotional eating or binge eating, in addition to containing the appetite-suppressing effects of bupropion. The idea behind Contrave is that by combining two medications in one pill, it will be more effective for weight loss than just Wellbutrin alone, but there haven't been any head-to-head trials comparing the two. Naltrexone can cause side effects that impair quality of life, including nausea, constipation, and dry mouth. There's also no generic version, so it's expensive—$525 for three months versus $10 for Wellbutrin, according to GoodRx (a website that offers medication price comparisons). And it's a twice-a-day pill. Hence it is not very popular for these reasons.

Adipex stimulates the central nervous system, which can reduce hunger cues and appetite. If you've been married, I equate its effects to how you feel on your wedding day. You may have felt so excited and amped up that it didn't even occur to you to eat, or another example is like the day you're making a big presentation at work and your nerves unsettle your stomach to the point that you just don't feel like sitting down and eating. It's thought that Adipex also works by indirectly increasing leptin levels, which makes you feel full, and decreasing the effects of neuropeptide Y, a neurotransmitter that stimulates the storage of fat and tamps down metabolism.

Pros: Relatively inexpensive, fairly effective, and easily obtained from online pharmacies. On average, people lose 5 percent of their body weight over three months. Adipex is a once-a-day pill (versus semaglutides, which must be injected, albeit only once a week or less if you're on a maintenance dose).

Cons: Imagine feeling like you're giving a huge presentation every day! Also, once you come off of the drug, it's very likely you'll gain the weight back. Because it is a stimulant, Adipex is not a good match for anyone with anxiety. Contrave has drug interactions that could lower the seizure threshold, so it should be avoided in anyone with a history of seizure disorder.

Qsymia also contains phentermine, the same stimulant that is in Adipex, and pairs it with topiramate, which is FDA-approved to prevent migraines and treat seizure disorders and has a side effect of promoting weight loss. The phentermine in Qsymia works by reducing appetite and suppressing food intake, while the topiramate helps you feel fuller longer and experience fewer cravings. As a result, Topamax (topiramate) alone has been evaluated in several studies for its potential as a weight loss treatment.[11]

Pros: Qsymia tends to be slightly more effective than Contrave. It's easy to use as it's a once-a-day pill.

Cons: Possible side effects include nausea, vomiting, dizziness, headaches, mood changes, and increased heart rate.

At-Home Remedies for Gaining Weight (for No Apparent Reason)

- Sufficient calories
- Sleep
- Not-too-intense exercise
- Hydration
- Protein and fiber
- Dog
- Psyllium
- Nutritionist
- Strength training

What You Can Do on Your Own to Manage Your Weight

Stop trying to undereat and overexercise. While small calorie deficits can be helpful in losing weight, starving yourself is not. I have patients who are eating fewer calories in a day than my toddler eats at breakfast, and doing intensive workouts several times a week, and they wonder why the weight won't budge. Or why the weight comes back on so quickly once they dial back the intense exercise or the focus on eating less. It's because eating too little cues your body to slow metabolism and hold on to every calorie it can.

I call this approach to losing weight "The Biggest Loser" model, after the weight-loss reality show of the same name that subjected its overweight participants to low-calorie diets and daily multi-hour workouts. It's based on the "calories in, calories out" model of weight loss that we've all been taught—if you want to lose weight, you have to eat less and move more. This approach has been shown to be misguided at best and harmful at worst, because losing weight via restricting calories (i.e., dieting) rarely leads to lasting weight loss. Once you step away from the diet, the weight tends to creep back on. Beyond that, dieting has been shown to result in a long-term slowing of metabolism. In fact, a study of former *The Biggest Loser* competitors found that they burned 30 percent fewer calories per day even years later, and most had regained at least most of the weight—some had gained so much weight that they were heavier than when they appeared on the show.[12]

Not only does dieting tend to not work, but it can create health risks of its own. The process of losing and then regaining weight, known as "weight cycling" in the scientific literature, has been found to be more harmful to your health than being overweight. Weight cycling has been linked to cardiovascular disease,[13] diabetes,[14] impaired immune function,[15] and metabolic dysfunction.

Keep an eye on your caloric consumption—maybe. For some women, it can be helpful to think in terms of calories, because there is a sweet spot of caloric intake for maintaining your weight or for dropping a few pounds if that's a priority for you. If you are trying to diet, it's tempting to dial your food intake back too far, which actually cues your metabolism to slow down. On the other hand, if you aren't thinking about how much you're eating, it's very easy to consume more calories than you need, especially in our current food culture, where portion sizes are bigger than ever. And not to mention the fact that so many of us are strapped for time that we reach for convenience foods that are engineered to be craveable, and because we are exhausted, we wash them down with sweetened coffee drinks and energy drinks, and then, boom, we can basically reach our daily calorie requirements in one meal.

To be clear, I am *not* suggesting that you dramatically restrict your food intake. But it can help to be mindful of how many calories you need and to give some thought to your food and drink choices so that you stay close to that number on most days. (There will always be days where feasting is absolutely appropriate!)

Most women require somewhere between 1,800 and 2,200 calories a day, and veering too far from this in either direction—either too few or too many—can mess with your metabolism in the long term. To figure out your basic calorie target, try the US Department of Agriculture's My Plate Plan (myplate.gov). It shows you how many calories you need to either lose a little weight or maintain your current weight based on your age, gender, height, weight, and activity level.

There is a huge caveat to this advice: If you've ever had any kind of disordered eating, or have become fixated on counting calories in the past, or fear that you might become stressed by trying to monitor your caloric intake, skip this tip. For some people, raising awareness and setting some basic parameters is helpful, but for others, it could be harmful to their mental or physical well-being, and that's not what we're after. When in doubt, drop the glass or two of wine a night.

Prioritize protein and fiber. Instead of thinking about "dieting," seek to include plenty of these two things that most of us are not eating enough of: protein and fiber. While these two types of foods won't address the endocrine disruption that's changing your metabolism, they will help counteract some of its negative effects.

I absolutely believe in eating all the macronutrients—proteins, carbs, and fats, and even a few sweets. I don't want you to eliminate any category of food; I just want you to make protein and fiber more of a focus. Think of them like a middle child—they're probably a little neglected, and spending a little effort to focus on them more will help the whole family flourish.

Protein is the primary building block of your body. Eating ample amounts—between 75 and 100 grams per day—helps counteract the loss of muscle tissue that starts accelerating in your forties and makes it easier to build muscle—which I'll talk about more specifically in the next tip—both of which help to keep your metabolic rate from slowing down. In addition, protein helps you feel full and keeps your blood sugar in a steadier range so that you crave fewer carbs. Think about it: Have you ever binged on chicken breasts or cottage cheese? I'm guessing the answer is no, because protein satisfies your appetite more quickly and fully than those things that are so easy to binge on, such as chips and pretzels.

Very few of my patients are eating enough protein when I first see them, because unless you are on the carnivore diet (which I don't recommend, as your body benefits from a wide variety of nutrients from a wide variety of foods), you have to consciously try to do so. In order to reach the target of 75 to 100 grams per day, or about 25 grams per meal, plus more in snacks. Every time you go to eat something, you want protein to be a primary component.

That means you want to have things on hand that are easy and quick to grab—cheese sticks, yogurt, cottage cheese, tuna in a pouch, nuts, seeds, and hard-boiled eggs, for example. Basically, you want to eat so much protein that you never want to hear the word again.

If you're a meat eater, keep it lean: turkey, chicken, and only the occasional red meat. Eggs provide about 7 grams per egg (so eat two). Fish and seafood are great options, as is dairy, whether that's cottage cheese, ricotta cheese, or plain yogurt (with a little honey or maple syrup if you don't like the taste of plain yogurt). Beans and legumes (adzuki beans, black beans, black-eyed peas, cannellini beans, chickpeas, edamame, great northern beans, green lentils, kidney beans, red lentils, pinto beans); nuts (almonds, pecans, walnuts, pistachios, cashews, macadamias, and nut butters); seeds (chia, flax, pumpkin, quinoa, sesame, sunflower; or tahini—which is ground sesame seeds); and protein powders (made from whey, peas, hemp, or collagen) are all your best friends.

Here's a list of foods that pack a decent amount of protein. Those with an asterisk are also good sources of fiber, since most women don't get enough fiber even though it's a key component of a healthy diet. Prioritize these starred foods and get even more bang for your buck.

HIGH-PROTEIN FOODS

Food	Protein Content	Serving Size
Cod	41 grams	½ a filet
Salmon	30.5 grams	½ a filet
Cottage cheese	28 grams	1 cup
Chicken breast	26.7 grams	½ of a full chicken breast
Turkey breast	25.6 grams	3 ounces
Lean beef	24.6 grams	3 ounces
Shrimp	20.4 grams	3 ounces
Greek yogurt	19.9 grams	7 ounces
Lentils*	18 grams	1 cup
Black beans*	17 grams	1 cup
Protein powder (on average—read label)	14–15 grams	1 scoop
Chickpeas*	14 grams	1 cup
Plain yogurt	11.9 grams	8 ounces
Pumpkin seeds*	8.8 grams	¼ cup
Milk	8.3 grams	1 cup
Quinoa*	8 grams	1 cup
Sunflower seeds*	7.25 grams	¼ cup
Peanut butter	7.2 grams	2 tablespoons
Eggs	6.3 grams	1 large egg
Cheese stick	6.3 grams	1 stick
Almonds*	6 grams	1 ounce
Pistachios*	5.7 grams	1 ounce
Chia seeds*	4.7 grams	2 tablespoons
Green peas*	4.3 grams	½ cup
Ezekiel bread (made from sprouted grains and legumes)*	4 grams	1 slice

Fiber helps reduce the higher glucose levels and insulin spikes that declining estrogen can trigger. Fiber is also super important for gut health—both to promote elimination and to feed your friendly gut bacteria. Like protein, fiber also helps you feel fuller for longer, so it helps prevent that hangry feeling that can cause you to reach for the easy, processed stuff that doesn't provide a lot of nutritional value. (Trader Joe's animal crackers, anyone? If you know, you know.) It has also been shown to help reduce heart disease, cholesterol, and diabetes.[16]

The goal for fiber intake is 25 grams per day, but the average woman is getting only about 10–15 grams per day. To reach the goal, aim to accompany the protein you're eating at every meal (you're doing that, right?) with some fruit and vegetables. Pears, apples, berries, and avocados are high-fiber choices. Fibrous vegetables include broccoli, brussels sprouts, butternut squash, carrots, green beans, kale, and sweet potatoes. Opt for whole grains (such as whole wheat bread and pasta, bean-based pasta, brown rice, steel-cut oats, and popcorn). As shown in the table above, many foods are rich in both protein and fiber—these are great foods to make your go-to choices. I sprinkle pumpkin or sunflower seeds on just about everything for a little extra protein and fiber. I also supplement with fiber gummies just to make sure.

While beefing up your fiber intake, it's important to drink plenty of water to keep that fiber moving through your digestive tract or you may experience bloating. If you haven't been eating much fiber, you'll want to add more into your diet gradually over the course of a few weeks—your digestive system will adjust.

Again, I'm including a chart of foods that are high in fiber so that you can start buying them on your trips to the grocery store and working them into your daily eating patterns. The asterisks indicate that these foods are good sources of protein, as well, killing two birds with one stone.

Eating plenty of protein and fiber will also help crowd out some of the emptier calories in your diet—the chips, bagels, and sweets. So, while eating more protein and fiber doesn't necessarily promote weight loss, it does help you get more of the nutrients your body needs to be healthy at any weight.

HIGH-FIBER FOODS

Food	Fiber Content	Serving Size
Lentils*	18 grams	1 cup
Black beans*	15 grams	1 cup
Artichoke hearts	14 grams	1 cup
Chickpeas*	12 grams	1 cup
Chia seeds*	9.8 grams	2 tablespoons
Butternut squash	7 grams	1 cup
Whole wheat pasta	7 grams	1 cup
Pears	6 grams	1 medium fruit
Almonds	6 grams	23 almonds
Ezekiel bread*	6 grams	1 slice
Pumpkin seeds*	5.2 grams	1 ounce
Oats	5 grams	1 cup
Kale (cooked)	5 grams	1 cup
Broccoli	5 grams	1 cup
Quinoa*	5 grams	1 cup
Avocado	5 grams	½ an avocado
Apples	4.5 grams	1 medium fruit
Raspberries	4 grams	½ cup
Green peas*	4.5 grams	½ cup
Asparagus	4 grams	1 cup
Brussels sprouts (cooked)	4 grams	1 cup
Edamame	4 grams	½ cup
Green beans (cooked)	4 grams	1 cup
Popcorn	4 grams	3 cups
Potato (russet)	4 grams	1 cup
Sweet potato	3.8 grams	1 medium sweet potato
Blackberries	3.75 grams	½ cup
Sunflower seeds (roasted)*	3.55 grams	¼ cup
Carrots (raw)	3.5 grams	1 cup

MY FAVORITE FIBER HACK

Yes, we all should eat more fiber-containing foods. But there's a pretty darn simple way to make sure you're hitting your daily fiber intake, and that's with an inexpensive and easy-to-take supplement—psyllium. This outer husk of the *Plantago ovata* plant forms a gel when combined with water, which bulks up your stool, regulates your elimination (it's helpful for both constipation and diarrhea), and does a host of other helpful things:

- Feeds your friendly gut bacteria, improving gut health
- Lowers LDL cholesterol (the bad kind)[17]
- Slows the release of glucose after eating, which helps moderate levels of blood sugar and insulin and has been shown to lower hemoglobin A1C[18]
- Helps you feel fuller longer, reducing appetite and eating to excess

The typical serving is a tablespoon, and while you can take it in capsule form, you may need to take a lot of capsules to reach this amount. I suggest buying the powder and stirring it into a glass of water (maybe add a splash of fruit juice for flavor), or even your first cup of coffee or tea, and then drinking it within a couple of minutes, as the psyllium husk can turn into gel pretty quickly.

Embrace strength training. In the first half of your life, you may have been able to drop a few pounds by working out more—probably something cardio-focused, like running, biking, spinning, or dance-based classes. Once you hit perimenopause, the weight-loss aspect of cardio doesn't really work in the same way, thanks to the underlying hormonal and metabolic changes discussed earlier in this chapter. To make matters worse, intense exercise can just perpetuate your stress levels during what's already a stressful time.

While moderate cardio—like brisk walking—is still a great thing to do because it strengthens your heart and has its own cascade of benefits (which I cover in chapter 9), it's not really going to help you with your belly fat. To counteract the tendency to accumulate extra fat around your waist that can happen in perimenopause, you really need to embrace strength training.

The driving force behind perimenopausal weight gain isn't that you have too much fat; it's more likely that you have too little muscle. That's where eating protein and lifting weights come in—they are the two sides of the same coin that are going to help you stave off more weight gain. And while strength training won't necessarily lead to weight loss—muscle weighs more than fat, after all—it can positively change your bodyweight composition to include more muscle and less fat, and that's a win. At the same time, strength training will help increase bone density, reduce your risk of falls and frailty in the decades to come, and keep your ratio of fat to muscle in a more balanced place. It also helps with the toned physique you may be looking for, although the number on the scale may go up, because again, muscle weighs more than fat. But don't be discouraged if that happens—if you are building muscle, you are getting healthier and building generational health.

Honestly, every perimenopausal person will benefit from weight training. Even if you're using a weight-loss medication, it's a nonnegotiable. (Be sure to read chapter 9 for more inspiration to make space for resistance training in your life; it's one of the four pillars of health I cover in that chapter.)

For now, know that your strength training does not have to be high-intensity CrossFit or involve barbells—it could be Pilates, yoga, or bodyweight exercises. I've also asked my trainer to put together three weight-training workouts you can do on your own, at home, even if you are a beginner (you can find them at heatherhirschmd.com/perimeno pause). Some of my patients express fears about growing too bulky or muscular if they start weight training. Let me tell you, you have to try very, very hard and eat a lot of excess protein to gain so much muscle that you bulk up. It's not something that will happen by accident.

Ideally, you'd do three strength-training workouts per week with a day of no strength training in between to give your muscles a chance to recuperate and rebuild. You can break it up by focusing on legs one day (doing things like squats and lunges), upper body and core another day (bicep curls, chest presses, knee push-ups), and full-body exercises (planks, burpees) on the third.

If you're new to strength training, there are lots of ways to get started. You can look for group classes at a gym; work with a personal trainer (some offer group classes, making it more cost-effective); or even find bodyweight routines on YouTube. Many gyms offer a free session with a trainer when you join, and it can be very helpful to have someone assess your current fitness, suggest a routine, and give you pointers on form.

Challenging your muscles and moving your body will also help address another driving factor behind perimenopausal weight gain: a lack of sleep. Nothing helps you conk out at night like moving your body while also challenging your brain (as strength training, with its attention to form and counting reps, can do). Weight training has also been shown to improve cognition and mood, based on the neuroplasticity (the formation of new thought patterns) involved in lifting weights.[19]

Build sleep-supportive habits. Although sleeping more won't necessarily help you lose weight, it will help you interrupt some of the underlying hormonal processes that are contributing to your weight gain. Try the "What You Can Do on Your Own" suggestions for improving sleep in chapter 4. Remember, strength training can also help you sleep better—and sleeping better will help you have the energy to lift heavy things.

Get beverage-savvy. If you want to curb weight gain, food isn't the only thing you need to think about consuming differently—you also need to think about what you're drinking, as beverages are a very common source of a large number of mostly empty calories.

In fact, the fourth-biggest source of calories in the American diet are soda, energy drinks, and sports drinks. And the biggest source of calories in these drinks is added sugar. The sixth-biggest category of calories is alcoholic beverages. (I talk more specifically about alcohol consumption in chapter 9.) Again, the "calories in, calories out" model of weight loss has been debated, but drinking one soda or one tall pumpkin spice latte and one glass of wine in a day adds about 300 calories while doing nothing to contribute to a feeling of fullness or to provide nutrients. Switching to sparkling water with a splash of juice or lemonade instead of soda, learning to love unsweetened coffee, and opting for another way to reduce your stress at the end of the workday instead of having a glass of wine can play an important role in stopping your upward weight gain trend.

Make sure you're staying hydrated by drinking sixty-four ounces (or eight glasses) of water per day. Your body can confuse thirst for hunger, so staying hydrated will help you avoid mindless eating. And being adequately hydrated promotes digestion, helps you feel fuller, and wards off fatigue and mood swings, both of which can otherwise cause you to reach for a snack to pep you up. You may have been able to skate by without thinking about how much water you've been drinking in your twenties and thirties, but now it's time to get a little more mindful about giving your body what it needs to feel its best. And one of those things is definitely water.

Get a dog. Okay, this may seem like a big step, but there is plenty of data that shows having a pet helps you maintain a healthy weight. After all, dogs don't walk themselves. Dog owners have been found to have fewer heart disease risk factors—in particular, their blood pressure tends to be lower than people who don't have dogs—and to fare better if they do experience a heart attack or stroke.[20] In addition, dog ownership can lower your stress, reduce loneliness, and bring more love into your life.[21] Of course, it's a big commitment at a time of your life when you may not have the bandwidth for any extra responsibilities. If you tell me you're too busy to get a dog, I believe you. But if it's something you've been considering—or your kids have been clamoring for—perhaps it could be a piece of the puzzle that helps you cope with the stress and the weight gain of perimenopause. (And remember, adopt, don't shop! There are so many loving and lovable dogs in shelters in need of a good home.)

Consider working with a nutritionist. This isn't technically something you do all on your own, but having an educated nutritional professional sit with you and help you assess your current diet, make changes that fit your lifestyle and preferences, and objectively assess your progress can be super helpful. This is an option if you're very motivated and understand that it's not a quick fix—it's about educating yourself about what works for your body and your health goals. A good nutritionist can also help with the components of emotional eating, such as eating to subconsciously cope with life stressors or as a measure of external comfort. It does take time and resources. For more of a DIY and likely affordable option, a digital weight-loss program such as Noom—which combines tools from cognitive behavioral therapy and access to human coaches with nutritional guidance—may be helpful.

I want to close this chapter with a story about a patient of mine that shows the power of shifting your focus away from how much you weigh and toward promoting whole-body health.

One of my patients, Leslie, entered her forties weighing 143 pounds. Around the age of forty-five, when her perimenopause really started kicking in, Leslie noticed that she was having trouble buttoning her jeans, even though she had cleaned up her diet by cutting way down on refined carbs, and she hadn't changed her exercise routine. By the time Leslie was forty-nine and in late perimenopause, she'd gained ten pounds. She was also experiencing low back pain that made it hard for her to keep up with the other women in her walking group, and she began having trouble staying asleep through the night because it was hard finding a comfortable position. The fatigue and the physical discomfort made exercising feel like a bridge too far.

Leslie tried going keto—and she did lose weight, although it came back once she started eating carbs again. Leslie chalked it all up to simply getting older and stress until her friends of similar ages started sharing their own stories of their various symptoms—including sleeping poorly and gaining weight seemingly out of nowhere. Leslie talked to her clinician about whether her various symptoms could be related to perimenopause, who told her (incorrectly) that her back pain sounded more like a musculoskeletal issue that was keeping her from exercise and thus leading to weight gain, and that she should try to get more sleep for her motivation. When Leslie asked about hormone therapy, her doc told her (also incorrectly, especially given that the symptoms she was experiencing were significantly impacting her quality of life) that the risks were too high.

Since it seemed like HT was off the table, Leslie decided to start strength training regularly—it was the first thing that helped reduce her back pain. And although it didn't help her lose weight, it did prevent her from gaining more. And she did feel stronger.

Once Leslie crossed over into menopause, other symptoms cropped up, including brain fog and a "nonexistent" (as she put it) libido. That's how she ended up in my office. Based on her symptoms, we started her on an estradiol patch and a nightly progesterone capsule. After she adjusted to these additions—and she started sleeping soundly through the night again—we added in a compounded testosterone cream for her libido. After a few months, Leslie started noticing muscle definition returning to her arms and shoulders and her jeans were no longer uncomfortable to button. Now, a few years past her menopause anniversary, Leslie feels great, her clothes fit, she's stronger, her back doesn't hurt, she's sleeping well, and she's interested in sex again. She still weighs a full ten pounds more than she did pre-perimenopause, but her cholesterol and A1C (a marker of blood glucose levels) and waist size are all in a healthy range—she and I both agree that she is in a great place even though she didn't technically "lose weight." She has expressed to me many times that she wishes when she first started suffering in perimenopause she had known what she knows today.

I share this story to remind you that the real goal is to feel good and tend to other markers of health, such as muscle mass and waist size, not to hit a certain number on the scale. If you're feeling bad about yourself because your weight isn't the number that you'd like it to be but your health is in a good place—stop and think about that. Do you really want to spend time feeling bad about yourself because your body is different than it once was? I say it's better to channel that energy toward building muscle, making sure you get the nutrients you need, getting the sleep you need to restore yourself, and appreciating your body as it is today.

CHAPTER 9

The Silent Symptoms

When Gail, a fifty-one-year-old accountant, was at her annual checkup, she could not recall the date of her last period when the medical assistant asked. Gail had been so busy with tax season that she completely forgot. After doing some quick thinking to jar her memory, Gail was shocked to realize that her last period was nine months ago. It left without a trace and seemingly never came back. She counted herself lucky to have not had noticeable symptoms like so many of her girlfriends had, but when her lab results come back, Gail was surprised to learn that her cholesterol was up by more than thirty points, even though her diet hadn't changed at all.

Some women, like Gail, are lucky to not experience perimenopausal symptoms until they are either well into their transition or they have blown past the one-year anniversary of their last period. If you are one of them, you're fortunate—but that doesn't mean your hormonal changes aren't impacting your current and future health.

Even if you don't experience a single noticeable symptom—the underpinnings of the health of every woman who goes through perimenopause are changing, and not for the better. The slow fade of estrogen has a direct impact on a laundry list of important health markers:

- Your cholesterol, glucose, and insulin levels tend to rise, which can then negatively impact your weight, heart health, metabolic health, and brain health and pave the way for type 2 diabetes, metabolic syndrome, fatty liver disease, and even dementia.

- Your bones are becoming less dense; your joints also feel the impact from the decline in estrogen, which could show up as a loss of range of motion, creakiness, or chronic pain. The loss in bone density, if left unchecked, often leads to osteoporosis and a high risk of fracture, which, for those who are in their seventies and beyond, can very often be fatal.

- You're losing muscle mass, which plays a role in your declining bone density (since what strengthens muscles also strengthens bones) and your slowing metabolism (as muscle tissue requires more calories to maintain than fat or bone). Not counteracting this natural loss of muscle paves the way for growing frail as you get older. We're also learning more and more about muscle's role in producing hormones and neurochemicals that have widespread effects throughout the body—even in the brain! If you have less muscle, you also have less of these helpful chemical messengers on hand, which has far-reaching ripple effects.

- Your vaginal and urinary tissues are becoming less resilient. While you may not necessarily notice this change in your daily life, you'll become more prone to urinary tract infections, sexually transmitted diseases, urinary incontinence, and even organ prolapse (where an abdominal organ can drop from its position and create a bulge in the vaginal canal).

SILENT SYMPTOMS AT A GLANCE

Hallmarks:

- Rising cholesterol
- Decreasing bone density
- Metabolic and weight changes (thanks to increasing blood sugar and insulin levels)

- Elevated blood pressure
- Declining muscle mass
- Loss of integrity in the vaginal and urinary tissues

Causative factors:

- Declining estrogen
- Declining testosterone

I don't want to scare you—these risks don't accumulate all at once. But I do want to alarm you just enough that you will be inspired to either start or continue doing the things that reduce these risks.

If you are reading this chapter because you want to get ahead of the curve and learn about perimenopause even though you aren't currently experiencing any symptoms, I want to give you a special shout-out—points for being proactive! (Your reading this book is also wise because, remember, perimenopause can last up to ten years; thus, while your symptoms may be silent now, they may get louder next year.)

I hope that even if you have identified a symptom set that is vexing you, you will read this chapter so that you understand the bigger health picture. By learning about the long-term health risks that perimenopause and menopause bring, you'll be better informed, which means you'll have the opportunity to make better choices. And you won't have to be blindsided in your sixties, like my patient Susan was. Susan, whose story I shared in my previous book, *Unlock Your Menopause Type*, considered herself one of the lucky ones—she never had hot flashes, or mood changes, or experienced painful sex. She thought menopause had taken it easy on her and was grateful for that fact, up until Thanksgiving Day when she was sixty-four. That's when Susan reached into the oven to pull out the turkey, heard a loud pop, and felt a sharp stab of pain in her lower back. Her trip to the ER revealed that she'd experienced a compression fracture and had osteoporosis—something she hadn't even realized she was at risk of. On top of her discomfort and shock, Susan felt betrayed by the medical system, as no doctor had ever warned her of the risk of osteoporosis, much less told her about the many preventive steps she could have taken to keep it at bay. That's why I call these symptoms silent—because you won't necessarily feel them happening. But just because they aren't making their presence known in this moment doesn't mean they aren't real.

Sometimes not having any symptoms can lull you into thinking you don't need to prioritize your self-care and health care. You may blow off scheduling your annual checkup or forget to book your screening tests because you feel fine. To prevent this from happening, I need to give you some tough love: Relying on youthful resilience and lucky genetics to keep your health in a good place is not a great long-term health strategy. At some point these changes mean you'll start going to the doctor more, perhaps needing more medications and experiencing more negative health events. Sorry to be a bummer, but this is not a drill.

The days of thinking you can "get away" with things—whether it's drinking too much, skimping on sleep, blowing off exercise, or opting for only highly processed foods—without paying any consequences are dwindling fast. It's time to admit that you soon will become the age where the music you listened to in middle school is playing on the oldies station. It's just part of the circle of life, and a sign that it's time to step it up.

I can't tell you how many postmenopausal women, like Susan, have come to me saying that they wish they had been given the facts about how their body would change during the menopause transition, wishing they could go back in time and make different decisions. It was only a few years ago that women simply didn't know about these risks. This is how we change that narrative.

The good news is that by learning about the health risks you face and the many things you can do to counteract them, you have an amazing opportunity to lay down a foundation now that will boost your health today and for decades to come. You have a huge opening for building what I call generational health for both yourself and the members of your family who come after you. Generational health is how you will be able to get down on the floor and play with your grandkids and how you can reduce the amount of time (and money) your children will need to devote to taking care of you. When you start adopting habits that support your long-term health—which I will cover in this chapter—in ten, twenty, or thirty years, you will be so grateful that you did.

Before we dive into the treatments and things you can do on your own, let's take a closer look at how the silent symptoms of perimenopause impact five primary areas of health: your heart, brain, bones, metabolic health, and genitourinary health. Because once you understand what's happening beneath the surface, your motivation to take steps to protect yourself will only increase.

Heart Health

I've said this before, but it bears repeating because too few people know and appreciate this startling fact: Cardiovascular disease is the leading cause of death for women. For much of our lives, we women have significantly lower rates of heart disease than men, but once we hit our fifties—when we are done menstruating—we catch up, and the loss of estrogen is a key factor. Research estimates that one out of every five US women die from heart disease.[1]

We don't know the direct causal link between declining estrogen and heart health, but we know a couple of factors: (1) Estrogen helps keep blood vessels healthy and pliable, which prevents high blood pressure and makes it easier for the heart to pump blood both to the body and back to the heart. High blood pressure, on the other hand, means the heart has to pump harder to keep blood circulating, which is why we docs like to keep a close eye on your blood pressure; (2) total cholesterol levels tend to increase through late perimenopause and into menopause, including higher LDL (the "bad" cholesterol) and triglycerides. This rise in cholesterol can be alarming because it tends to jump 10 to 15 percent, or about 10 to 20 milligrams per deciliter—even if you're eating little to no red meat and plenty of vegetables.[2]

While there isn't clear data that says hormone therapy prevents the diagnosis of hypertension or dyslipidemia (the medical term for high cholesterol), data does show that women who take HT within ten years from their last period are less likely to die from cardiovascular events and have a lower risk of heart attacks.[3] The link is clear enough in the research that the American Heart Association (AHA) came out with a paper in 2020 officially declaring that menopause is an independent risk factor for heart disease,[4] stating, "The reported findings underline the significance of the menopause transition as a time of accelerating cardiovascular disease risk, thereby emphasizing the importance of monitoring women's health during midlife, a critical window for implementing early intervention strategies to reduce cardiovascular risk." Coming from such a mainstream medical organization, this AHA statement was groundbreaking.

Metabolic Health

When you're in your thirties and forties it's easy to take your metabolic health—an umbrella term that refers to your glucose and insulin levels, your weight, and your risk of diabetes as well as some of the measures of heart health, including low-density cholesterol levels, blood pressure, and triglyceride levels—for granted. Sure, you might eat more sweets than you should, but you likely aren't yet thinking about how that might be impacting your blood sugar levels over time. Or you might be thinking that an increased risk of diabetes is something your mom needs to worry about, but you don't because you are still young.

Perimenopause changes all that—as estrogen declines, our measures of metabolic health tend to trend downward with it. Now is the time to start keeping tabs on five indicators of metabolic health: waist circumference; triglyceride levels (a type of fat that circulates in the blood); high-density lipoprotein levels (or HDL, aka the "good" kind of cholesterol); blood pressure; and fasting blood sugar levels (refer back to the sidebar "Metabolic Syndrome and Perimenopause" in chapter 1 for the levels you want to stay under). If three of the values of these five criteria creep into unhealthy ranges, you officially have what's known as metabolic syndrome, or a cluster of conditions that collectively indicate an increased risk of diabetes, stroke, and heart disease.

While both men and women in the United States experience metabolic syndrome in similar numbers (approximately 37 percent of American adults have it), its rates are rising more quickly in women than in men (we went from a prevalence of 31.7 percent in 2011 to 36.6 percent in 2016).[5] It is extremely important for perimenopausal women to look out for and safeguard against metabolic syndrome. Declining estrogen contributes directly to it, as lower estrogen can trigger the accumulation of belly fat and an expanding waistline. Since estrogen plays a role in regulating blood sugar, when there is less of it on hand, your blood sugar tends to stay higher, contributing to your risk of diabetes and to the storage of fat, particularly around the waist.

Brain Health

The scary truth is that about one in five women will develop dementia, and women make up two-thirds of dementia patients. Like any chronic disease, dementia has many contributing factors, including heart health (because if your heart has trouble pumping blood, your brain will get less blood flow and, therefore, less oxygen and fewer nutrients); diet (as inflammatory foods and sugar have both been found to be detrimental to brain health); toxic exposures; and lack of sleep, to name a few. Because the brain is ripe with estrogen receptors and estrogen is anti-inflammatory, it is thought that estrogen's decline can be a source of neuroinflammation. This likely explains why brain fog is a common perimenopausal symptom—as estrogen becomes volatile, cognitive function can take a hit. Eighty percent of women regain their sharp and usual cognitive function after their hormones stabilize into later menopause. But for 20 percent of us, the long tentacles of dementia—a disease that may take decades to develop—start to take root.

DISCERNING THE DIFFERENCE BETWEEN COGNITIVE DECLINE AND PERIMENOPAUSAL BRAIN FOG

Is it perimenopause? Or is it early-onset Alzheimer's? This is a question many of my patients confess to worrying about. Here is a quick primer on how to tell the difference between the two. Refer back to chapter 6 for more detail about the symptoms and strategies for addressing brain fog—as well as more detail about the difference between it and dementia.

Symptoms of perimenopausal brain fog: Trouble finishing tasks, difficulty finding the right word, challenges with concentration (such as reading a book or finishing a spreadsheet), short-term memory lapses (why did I walk into this room?), misplacing items

Red flags of potential cognitive decline: Forgetting your way home, forgetting names of your nuclear family, forgetting what day or time of year it is, forgetting your anniversary or other important dates, displaying poor judgment that continues or gets worse

---

Bone Health

In the head-to-toe tour we took of estrogen's effects in chapter 1, we covered that the lessening of estrogen also cues an acceleration in the loss of bone density, and that women are more likely to experience a broken bone due to osteoporosis than they are to suffer from a cardiovascular event, a stroke, and a diagnosis of breast cancer combined. Beyond osteoporosis, women also experience an increase in osteoarthritis (which women are significantly more likely than men to experience), joint pain, and musculoskeletal pain, as well as a loss of lean muscle mass. We now refer to this as the musculoskeletal syndrome of menopause. All of these conditions can progress and significantly impair your quality of life if left unattended or undiscussed (a possibility we are reducing with this book, thank you very much).

Genitourinary Health

There are so many possible changes during this time to your genitourinary tract—which covers everything from the clitoris, vulva, and vagina to the bladder—that they have their own name: the genitourinary syndrome of menopause (GSM). (And if you think that name is scary-sounding, it used to be called vaginal atrophy!)

For all the reasons I outlined in the tour of the body in chapter 1, perimenopause kicks off a fundamental change in the integrity of the tissues in your genitourinary tract as well as the pH level of those tissues, which can result in a host of negative developments, including vaginal and vulvar dryness that can cause discomfort throughout the day and pain during intercourse; a lack of blood flow that can reduce arousal, sensitivity, and the ability to orgasm; abnormal Pap smear results; urinary incontinence; frequent urinary tract infections; an increased susceptibility to sexually transmitted disease; a weakened pelvic floor; and organ prolapse. While it's highly unlikely you'll experience all these things, it's very probable that you will experience more than one.

It is my sincere hope that you'll let these insights motivate you to commit some time, energy, and even a little money when you can swing it toward taking care of yourself. I know you likely have a lot of other people depending on you, and that you have a growing list of things to take care of, and you might be feeling like there isn't much left over to devote to self-care—or that "self-care" is a loaded term that sounds frivolous or like a privilege. Here's my response to that thought process: Not only do you deserve to feel good in your body and enjoy a high quality of life, but you have the potential to save yourself a lot of expense (in health-care costs and lost work) and discomfort (from your symptoms and potential treatments). If you think you can't afford to tend to your health, think about it this way: You can't afford *not* to. Thankfully, all of these silent symptoms and an increase in disease risk can be avoided with one basic approach, and that is tending to your four pillars of health:

- Sleep
- Diet
- Exercise
- Mental health

These are the daily choices, habits, and attitudes that not only help you feel your best, but also help your body function at its best both in the short term—so that you have more energy and are more resilient— and the long term—so that you become less susceptible to the chronic diseases and conditions that become more and more common with age. When you take good care of these four basic areas, your body can take of you.

As helpful as hormone therapy and other medical treatments can be—and I will cover these at the end of the chapter—your most powerful strategy for remedying the silent symptoms of perimenopause is to build good habits that support these four pillars of health. These habits are things that every woman who wants to build generational health needs to embrace now.

Of these, the pillar I recommend you start with—unless it's already in a good place—is sleep, because without getting sufficient rest, it's a lot harder to take care of your other three pillars, and with it, everything else flows more easily.

Pillar #1: Sleep

Women need more sleep than men, and we are less likely to get it. Although women tend to sleep about eleven minutes longer than men at every life stage, they also experience more fragmented sleep than men.[6] In fact, women are 40 percent more likely to experience insomnia than men.[7]

Sleep has the biggest beneficial impact on everything—your mood, your energy levels, your bandwidth for exercise and making healthy food choices, your stress, and even your appetite, as a poor night's sleep can increase levels of ghrelin—a hormone that stimulates your appetite—and lower levels of leptin—a hormone that makes you feel full.[8]

Impaired sleep is also hard on your heart: both sleeping fewer than seven hours per night and experiencing multiple awakenings in the night have been shown to increase the risk of stroke, heart attack, and myocardial infarction.[9] Impaired sleep isn't great for your brain, either. While there isn't yet an established link between poor sleep in your forties and dementia risk later, the sleep habits you strengthen now are likely to continue, and once you reach your fifties, research has shown that sleeping six hours or less increases the risk of developing dementia by 30 percent.[10]

Perimenopause may also increase your risk of developing sleep apnea—a condition we discussed in the previous chapter—because estrogen can weaken the tissues of your airways and perimenopausal weight gain can press on your upper airways when you're lying down. This is problematic because sleep apnea is a known risk factor for heart disease and dementia. If you have any of the symptoms listed in the "Sleep Apnea Warning Signs" section, don't delay; talk to your clinician about it. She will likely order a sleep study, which may require you to spend the night in a sleep clinic, although there are at-home tests available now.

SLEEP APNEA WARNING SIGNS

- Your partner or roommate tells you you're snoring loudly, especially with pauses and gasps for air
- You toss and turn frequently while sleeping
- Persistent daytime sleepiness
- Dry mouth
- Morning headaches

If you don't already have good sleep habits, now is the time to dial them in—and avoid developing bad ones.

How do you do that exactly? If you have not yet read chapter 4, flip back there to review the list of sleep hygiene strategies I outline. In brief, there are many simple and effective ways to boost your sleep tonight—it *can* get better.

Pillar #2: Exercise

Exercise is a crucial piece of your health strategy—it's about so much more than looking good in your bathing suit. Exercise has quite an impressive and comprehensive list of benefits for targeting the very things that perimenopause and menopause make us more vulnerable to.

- Exercise helps lower glucose and insulin levels by cuing the body to move glucose out of the bloodstream and into the muscles, where it can be used for energy. This means movement will help to counteract the blood sugar and insulin disruptions that can occur as estrogen declines—thus it will help you avoid developing metabolic syndrome.
- Exercise is a powerful mood booster. It triggers the release of many different chemicals, including endorphins, dopamine, and other neurotransmitters that help to reduce stress and give you mild feelings of euphoria. Some types of movement, like yoga, Pilates, and tai chi, are also mindfulness in motion because you really have to focus on where your body is in space, which is also calming.
- Endorphins are also natural painkillers, making those perimeno-pausal aches and pains less pronounced; also, making your muscles stronger takes pressure off your joints, which alleviates potential sources of chronic pain.
- Exercise cues your bones to get stronger—a great counterbalance to the natural loss in bone density that tends to accelerate during late perimenopause and into menopause.

- Exercise strengthens your heart muscle and improves circulation, meaning every cell in your body gets more of the life-giving oxygen and nutrients that are delivered by your blood. And, exercise raises good cholesterol and lowers triglycerides while also lowering blood pressure—all of which means that exercise is a great insurance policy against cardiovascular disease.

- Exercise is also great for your brain—walking as little as thirty-eight hundred steps a day has been found to lower dementia risk by 25 percent; brisk walking (at a pace of 112 steps per minute) for just thirty minutes per day, even if those thirty minutes don't happen all at once, was found to reduce the risk of developing dementia by 62 percent.[11] And your muscles produce many brain chemicals, including brain-derived neurotrophic factor (BDNF), which cues the formation of new neurons in the brain and new connections between existing neurons, so as you build muscle, you also build your brain. How's that for a bonus? Plus, as we covered when we talked about heart health earlier in this chapter, the increased circulation that exercise triggers means your brain also gets more nutrients and oxygen.

- Exercise helps you ward off weight gain.

- Exercise helps you get to sleep faster and stay asleep for longer (as long as you don't work out within three hours of bedtime, when it could stimulate you enough that it actually impedes your sleep). So, if you've started trying to improve your sleep but have had only marginal success, try prioritizing exercise and see if it naturally helps you sleep better.

Really, no matter how much you are already moving—or not moving—you probably ought to be finding ways to work even more movement into your life. Notice that I said "more movement," not "more intense exercise." While, yes, you do want to do some formal exercise— and I'll give you a tour through the types that are most important for you to incorporate in just a moment—you also just want to move more in general, and not necessarily by doing things that push your limits. Running errands on foot, taking mini movement breaks throughout your workday, or doing a few stretches on the floor while you watch a show are all beneficial.

Moderate exercise—so that you work up a light sweat and can hold a conversation, although your breath may be noticeable—is really all it takes to reap the benefits of exercise I just listed. In fact, pushing harder than that can be stressful to the body. I used to love CrossFit, but I don't do it much anymore because I noticed that I felt very sore and wiped out after the workouts. If you live for CrossFit, I'm not going to tell you to stop, but pay attention to how your body reacts to it—if you notice you're catching every virus, getting injured, or just feeling worn-down, your body may be telling you that it could use something a little less intense.

There are three basic categories of exercise:

- Strength training
- Cardio
- Balance/flexibility

I have many patients who tend to do only one kind of exercise— perhaps they are runners, but never stretch or lift weights; or they are devoted to yoga but never do anything to work up a sweat. Ideally, you'll do some exercises in each category on a regular basis. Let's take a peek at what that looks like.

Strength Training

Types of exercises: Things like push-ups and squats where you use your body weight for resistance; using dumbbells or resistance training machines to perform exercises like bicep curls and deadlifts; or using resistance bands. (You can access one beginner-friendly workout using each type of weight at heatherhirschmd.com/perimenopause.)

Benefits: Strength training is especially important for bone health, reducing frailty and falls as you get older, brain health, protecting your joints, maintaining a healthy weight (by raising your overall metabolic rate), regulating blood sugar, boosting mood, and, yes, building muscle.

How often: Ideally, you'll do some kind of strength training two or three times a week, with a day off from lifting in between each workout so that your muscles have a chance to recover.

If you are going to do just one form of exercise, choose strength training, which I consider to be nonnegotiable for perimenopausal and menopausal women because it is so important for maintaining muscle mass and bone density. It can also perform a double duty: If you do whole-body exercises, like lunges while holding a light dumbbell over your head, that also counts as cardio.

Moderate Cardio

Types of exercises: Anything that gets your heart rate up is technically considered cardio, including walking, jogging, dancing, biking, rowing, riding the cardio machines at the gym, playing a sport like tennis, basketball, or soccer, and even whole-body strength-training moves, like burpees.

Benefits: Moderate cardio strengthens your heart, lungs, and circulatory system, increases circulation, regulates blood sugar levels, protects your brain against dementia, strengthens bones, reduces stress, boosts digestion, increases the capacity of your muscles, strengthens your immune system, improves sleep, and enhances mood.

How often to do the exercises: Two to three times a week for at least thirty minutes total (you can break it up into smaller chunks if necessary). You want to be working at a level where you are breaking a light sweat but can still carry on a conversation, although your breath may be noticeable. (If you're talking to a friend on the phone, they will wonder what you're doing.) And even on days when you're not doing official cardio, work in as many movement snacks as you can feasibly do—doing a few lunges or squats for a break, walking up and down the stairs—to help keep your muscles loose, refresh your mind, and give your heart a little boost. It all counts.

If you were going to choose just one form of cardio to commit to, walking is a fabulous choice, no matter how much time you have or how fit you are. It's not only good for your heart, but it's great for your mental health to get outside in the natural light, breathe the fresh air, and see the natural sights (even if it's just the sky and the clouds because you live in an urban area with little vegetation). Nothing clears my mind better than taking a twenty-minute walk.

There are ways to make your cardio tick a lot of boxes. Taking a fitness class is a great opportunity to meet new people and perhaps learn something new. Walking or biking with a friend is a great way to get social time. Signing up for a race or other challenge will give you a meaningful goal and a sense of purpose.

Flexibility and Balance

Types of exercise: Yoga, stretching, Pilates, tai chi, barre

Benefits: Reduces muscular tension, supports joint health and range of motion, raises spatial awareness to improve balance and posture, promotes proper alignment and wards off chronic aches and pains and headaches, prevents injuries, reduces stress, and promotes mindfulness

How often to do the exercises: Once or twice a week

These forms of mindfulness in motion are so good for your overall well-being, and they touch parts of health that strength training and cardio just can't—things like posture, alignment, flexibility, and mindfulness. Whether you go to a class, practice on your own at home, or find a creator on YouTube or an app, these pursuits are how you tend to entire embodiment.

Pillar #3: Diet

Now is the time to adopt eating habits that will provide a foundation for health and help prevent any silent symptoms from developing into a full-blown condition or disease. The general eating pattern that has been shown to promote health most consistently is a Mediterranean-style diet with plenty of plant-based protein, lean animal proteins (including fish), fruits, vegetables, whole grains, and healthy fats. Basically, the diet consists of eating primarily whole foods with sparing sweets; little saturated fat (from animal products such as bacon and red meat); and minimal ultra-processed foods (like chips, cookies, and bars).

This is also the perfect time to take a look at the beverages you're consuming regularly to make sure they aren't a source of empty calories—whether from soda, energy drinks, sweetened coffee drinks, or alcoholic beverages (I talk more specifically about alcohol later in this chapter).

As the loss of estrogen generally means your cells and tissues become drier, it's more important that you prioritize drinking plenty of filtered water so that you stay hydrated. In addition to being necessary for keeping every system of your body working optimally, hydration helps with concentration, energy, and keeping fatigue and headaches at bay.

Protein

I'm listing protein first because, from here on out, your protein needs only continue to increase. Once you reach your thirties, you start losing muscle mass—up to 5 percent per decade, and that starts to really accumulate and pick up steam once you're in your fifties and sixties. There are two prongs to maintaining muscle and strength as you age—exercise and diet. Because everyone needs to eat but not everyone exercises (although I hope I will convince you to do so), supporting your muscle mass through diet is absolutely vital, and the way you do that is by eating ample amounts of protein.

For guidelines on which protein-rich foods to add to your diet and how to make sure you're getting enough, refer to the "What You Can Do on Your Own" section in chapter 8, about the "Gaining Weight for No (Apparent) Reason" symptom set. Even if you aren't interested in losing weight, you need to eat more protein.

Complex Carbohydrates

Carbs are your body's friend, as long as they are complex carbs, which means they naturally contain decent amounts of fiber. Because it is so beneficial for gut health, digestion, and heart health (because fiber helps bind excess cholesterol and keep your blood lipids in a good place), you want to be getting 25 grams of fiber per day—a number very few Americans are reaching.

Prioritizing complex carbs can go a long way toward coming closer to that fiber target. They include most vegetables and fruit, whole grains, and legumes (although because legumes are also rich in plant-based protein, I included them in the protein category). Right alongside the protein you want to eat at every meal, you want plenty of vegetables— dark leafy greens, cruciferous vegetables (like broccoli, brussels sprouts, cauliflower, and radishes), and deeply hued vegetables (like eggplant, peppers, sweet potatoes, and tomatoes). Fruit makes a great snack or dessert (especially when you have it with some cheese, yogurt, nuts, or nut butter). Because some fruit can be high in sugar and low in fiber— like bananas, grapes, and mangoes—stick to lower-sugar, higher-fiber options, like apples, berries, citrus, and stone fruits for the most part. And of course, complex carbs include whole grains like brown rice, steel-cut oats, and whole wheat bread—servings of these should be one cup of rice or oats; one thick or two thin slices of whole wheat bread.

For more specific guidance on getting sufficient amounts of fiber, refer to the "What You Can Do on Your Own" section of chapter 8.

Fats

No diet is complete without ample healthy fat. Fat helps your body absorb nutrients, protects your organs, makes up a large portion of your brain, and sheathes your nerves. The trick is to choose the right kind of fat—primarily, that means more unsaturated fats (mostly from plants) and fewer saturated fats (from animals, such as fatty meats, butter, and lard) or damaged fats (such as fried foods, which are cooked in oil that's been heated to high temperatures that degrade the fats).

Healthy fats include avocado, avocado oil, fatty fish such as salmon, nuts, nut butters, olives, and olive oil. Aim to eat two to three servings of fat each day. And aim to eat fatty fish two or three times a week, as the omega-3 fatty acids it contains help reduce triglycerides and increase HDL (the good cholesterol) levels, and reduce the risk of blood clots and developing heart arrythmias as well. I personally never leave the grocery store without a bag of small avocados and, thanks to my Italian American upbringing, I tend to pour olive oil on everything.

And then, no matter what you're eating, allow yourself to not do anything else while you're eating, except perhaps talking with the people you might be eating with, so that you can savor the taste and be mindful of how your body is feeling as you're eating. This promotes relaxation and thus digestion. It can also make eating nourishing for your soul as well as your body.

I know it's a challenge to dial in healthy eating—I struggle with it myself. I have tried meal planning and prepping and I know it's hard to keep up. My best advice is to simplify—find your favorite meals and snacks and then stick with them until you need to change things up again to suit your palate and your desire for novelty. Keep things fresh by swapping in different vegetables, fruits, and herbs that are in season—for example, have steel-cut oats with some chopped nuts and apples in the fall, and plain yogurt with peaches or berries in the summer. This way, you can have your shopping and meal prep on autopilot for a little while. For novelty's sake, try a meal kit service, or try things you don't prepare at home when you go out.

A Frank Look at the Health Risks of Alcohol

While we're talking about diet, I want to take a moment to discuss one particular type of beverage—alcohol.

We live in a culture that normalizes drinking alcohol. Even in the health community, a daily glass or two of red wine is believed to have health benefits as it is often part of the traditional Mediterranean diet, which is widely heralded as one of the healthiest eating patterns in the world. But I don't think we balance out the conversation by talking enough about the health risks of alcohol.

I find it interesting that for twenty years we warned women off taking hormone therapy in menopause because one study found that doing so could cause eight additional cases of breast cancer in every ten thousand women (which is what the WHI initially reported in 2002), when at the same time, research has clearly shown that drinking more than one glass of alcohol per day is linked to an additional 27.86 cases of breast cancer per ten thousand women.[12] So why do doctors scare women about estrogen use but don't talk about alcohol? I also find it interesting that we have (rightly) scared people off smoking cigarettes and doing illicit drugs, but we haven't had widespread public awareness campaigns about the dangers of alcohol.

I'm not saying to not ever drink any alcohol. But I am saying that there are risks to drinking alcohol that we don't talk about or factor in enough. Alcohol is a known carcinogen, for starters. According to the American Society of Clinical Oncology, alcohol is causally associated with cancer of the larynx, esophagus, liver, colon, and breast.[13] The cancer risk of having one or fewer drinks per day may be small, but they are still real—in a 2024 report, the US surgeon general, Dr. Vivek Murthy, released an advisory on the risks of alcohol. In that report, Murthy shared that alcohol is responsible for twenty thousand of the deaths from cancer in the US each year, and for 16.4 percent of all incidences of breast cancer in the US.[14] And the risks rise the more you drink.

Also, alcoholic beverages do contain calories, and if they contain fruit juice, sugar, or soda (which most cocktails do), they are highly caloric. Yet I have seen so many women in my practice who are careful to eat healthfully and exercise yet wonder why they're still gaining weight when they are drinking at least two drinks multiple times a week. Cutting out the alcohol is probably the missing step.

Finally, alcohol is a known sleep disruptor—because it is a depressant, when you sober up you also get relatively more energized, which can wake you up. And sleep is already likely to be disrupted in perimenopause.

There are many things you can do for your health, but drinking a glass of wine really isn't one of them. Yes, red wine has antioxidants in it, but so do berries, peppers, and olive oil (among many other foods). The problem with having just one glass of wine is that after you have that one glass, it gets harder to resist the urge to pour yourself a second glass, and maybe even a third. Don't even get me started on mommy wine culture, which essentially makes a joke out of how hard it is to be a mom, and how that difficulty is best dealt with by pouring yourself a glass (or maybe hiding it in a sippy cup). I get it (trust me, I have three children); it is really hard to be a mom, but engaging in risky behavior really won't make it easier.

I hope that looking at the data will help counteract the collective embrace of alcohol as just a part of regular life, and inspire you to start thinking about how much and how often you drink.

To help you objectively assess how much you're drinking, the Dietary Guidelines for Americans suggest that women limit their alcohol consumption to one drink per day, with a drink defined as:

- 12 fluid ounces (355 milliliters) of beer;
- 5 fluid ounces (148 milliliters) of wine; or
- 1.5 fluid ounces (44 milliliters) of hard liquor.

These serving sizes are often smaller than the typical drink. If you are having your drink at a restaurant, for example, a pint of beer contains sixteen ounces, and the typical glass of wine is six ounces—although some restaurants offer a nine-ounce option—and a standard margarita contains two ounces of tequila plus a splash of a liqueur such as triple sec or Grand Marnier. At home, it's hard to know how many ounces of wine you're pouring yourself unless you pour it into a measuring cup first.

I know many women enjoy their glass of wine and can drink it thoughtfully. I also understand that a glass of wine can help us feel more relaxed, a little freer, maybe a little happier—it's for these reasons that it's all too easy to use alcohol to mask any unpleasant emotion or distract us from parts of our lives that may need attention. But I encourage you to check in with yourself to assess how much you're drinking, and why. Some of those reasons may be to reduce stress, or to go along with social norms, to fall asleep, or to get in the mood for sex. Whatever reason you discover, ask yourself what else you could do to achieve the same ends. If you make the effort to be more thoughtful about your choice to drink— or not drink—you may very well open the door to making choices that are more aligned with aging vitally and gracefully without the dangers associated with alcohol intake.

Pillar #4: Mental Health

Mental health is an inseparable facet of health. Your mood plays a huge role in your quality of life, your relationships, and each decision you make—including those about what you'll do, or not do, to take care of yourself. Because perimenopause can contribute to mental health symptoms such as anxiety or depression, and because midlife can be an inherently stressful time of life where your responsibilities are at an all-time high, you'll want to take a proactive approach to keeping your headspace positive.

Take some time to think about what helps you feel your best mentally. Is it journaling? Making sure you connect with friends so that you can vent and feel heard (and support them, which also gives you a boost)? Meditating or doing breathing exercises? Prioritizing gratitude? Affirmations? Therapy? All of the above? Whatever your unique prescription is, think about not only what you'll do but also when and how you'll do it.

I know that it's easy for a physician to say, "Reduce your stress," and quite another thing to actually do it. But there truly is no other time of life when you need these tools and strategies more, even though you may very likely feel too busy to implement them. You need productive coping skills now, not when life calms down (because, truth time: It won't). Without thinking about your mental health plan, you'll be too likely to reach for coping mechanisms that only make you feel worse, whether that's drinking wine, picking fights, or going down a negative thought spiral.

I myself have recently started seeing a therapist again—I find cognitive behavioral therapy to be immensely helpful and recommend it to patients regularly—and I am a big fan of the guided meditations and teachings of Dr. Joe Dispenza. I've rededicated myself to getting some form of exercise as many days of the week as I can manage because it helps me turn my attention from whatever is stressing me out and toward how I'm feeling in my body and what my body is doing in the moment. Especially weight training. Nothing is better than feeling yourself physically grow stronger.

Know that tending to the other three pillars also plays a huge role in mental health—sleep helps you process memories and refresh mentally; eating well prevents blood sugar spikes and crashes that can take your mood on a roller coaster, provides the nourishment your brain needs to function, and feeds your friendly gut bacteria, which produce many neurotransmitters; and exercise is a great way to blow off steam as well as trigger the production of neurochemicals that keep your brain happy and resilient.

Regarding all four of the pillars, I encourage you to follow up with a provider when these strategies don't feel like enough. This could be your primary care physician, your Menopause Society certified practitioner (MSCP), or a specialist such as a personal trainer, nutritionist, sleep medicine doctor, or licensed therapist. Yes, it may require you to spend some money and some time, but remember, you are trying to build generational health that will not only support you throughout the next several decades but also positively influence your family now and into the future, too. I think of it this way: Spend it now and live a longer, healthier life; or spend more later and have a reduced quality of life. Just like investing money in a retirement account, the earlier you start, the bigger the payoff you'll experience later.

Four Pillars Check-In

As important as it is to learn what you can do to support your pillars of health, merely expanding your knowledge isn't going to create meaningful change in your life. Use this simple self-assessment to see which of the pillars need your attention the most, celebrate what's already going well, and make a game plan of exactly which strategies and tools you'll implement in order to move those ratings closer to ten. Write your answers in a journal or on your phone's Notes app.

Sleep
- On a scale of 1 to 10, how is your sleep?
- List what's going well.
- List what you'd like to do better.
- Name three specific things you'd like to try to raise that score.

Diet
- On a scale of 1 to 10, how is your diet?
- List what's going well.
- List what you'd like to do better.
- Name three specific things you'd like to try to raise that score.

Exercise
- On a scale of 1 to 10, how is your exercise?
- List what's going well.
- List what you'd like to do better.
- Name three specific things you'd like to try to raise that score.

Mental Health
- On a scale of 1 to 10, how is your mental health?
- List what's going well.
- List what you'd like to do better.
- Name three specific things you'd like to try to raise that score.

Treatments That Can Help (in the Order I Typically Recommend Them)

You may be wondering, *Should I start hormone therapy preemptively even if I'm not currently experiencing bothersome symptoms?* There is no solid data (yet) that says starting HT in perimenopause has long-term health benefits (however, there is data to show that HT can prevent chronic disease when started within ten years after a woman's last menstrual period, so as you can see, it's a bit tricky with perimenopause). HT is still recommended—and FDA-approved—only to treat certain symptoms, although one of these is loss of bone density, which we know every perimenopausal woman faces. If you truly have no symptoms, then there might not be a clear reason to start HT preemptively. Although, if you have had a DXA scan that shows you already have osteopenia, you may strongly consider preemptive HT. DXA scans aren't officially recommended until age sixty-five, but if anyone in your family has suffered a broken hip, or you smoke, consume excessive alcohol, have a low body weight, had an eating disorder or a condition that could interfere with nutrient absorption such as celiac disease, or are taking medications including glucocorticoids, aromatase inhibitors, or gonadotropin-releasing hormone agonists, which can compromise bone density, had a very early perimenopause, or have hyper- or hypothyroidism, talk to your doctor about ordering one for you.

You still can—and should—talk to your doctor to ask questions about when they recommend starting HT, and plan for the months and years ahead. Remember, your symptom situation could look very different even six months from now.

The treatments I do tend to recommend to patients who don't yet have noticeable symptoms, although they are in their forties and so very likely on the perimenopause on-ramp, include:

A **progesterone-releasing IUD,** as it protects against uterine cancer, prevents an unintended pregnancy, and can also decrease the amount of cramping and bleeding you experience with each cycle.

Low-dose oral contraceptives to keep your cycle predictable, lessen bleeding, and make your hormone levels more stable. This classification of medications also prevents against unintended pregnancies and can reduce acne and hair growth in unwanted places by lowering androgen (testosterone) levels.

Local vaginal estrogen can be used preventively to help protect against developing vaginal dryness, pain with intercourse, or recurrent urinary tract infections.

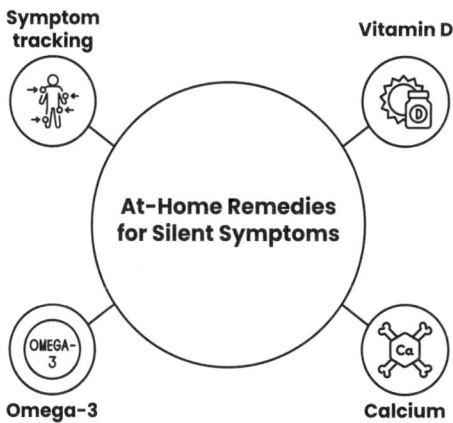

Symptom tracking

Vitamin D

At-Home Remedies for Silent Symptoms

Omega-3

Calcium

What You Can Do on Your Own for the Silent Symptom Set

In addition to tending to your four pillars of health, now is also the perfect time to:

Start tracking your period and your symptoms. This is the best way to understand where you are in your perimenopause transition. In addition to writing down any symptoms you may experience, note if your periods are getting longer or shorter, heavier or lighter, and if cramping is increasing or decreasing.

Get your vitamin D levels checked by your clinician and take enough as a supplement to get your levels to at least 30 nmol/L at a minimum. If your levels are under 30 nmol/L, start taking 1,000—2,000 IUs daily of over-the-counter vitamin D, then have your levels checked again in twelve weeks to see if you are absorbing it.

Prioritize omega-3 fatty acids, which help reduce inflammation and decrease the risk of cardiovascular disease while also supporting brain health. (I also cover omega-3s in the "What You Can Do on Your Own" section of chapter 5—refer back to it for food sources and supplement guidance.)

Aim to get 1,200 mg of calcium a day, from a combination of diet and supplementation, to protect against the decline in bone density that naturally occurs as estrogen levels lower.

PART III

SET YOURSELF UP FOR SMOOTH MENOPAUSAL SAILING

CHAPTER 10

Targeted Treatments for Solo Symptoms

While many perimenopausal symptoms occur in clusters, there are many others that ride solo and can pop up at different times during transition. (What can I say? Perimenopause is a gift that keeps on giving.)

In this chapter, I'll cover the strategies that can mitigate some of these solo symptoms, and also provide some insight as to why they may be occurring in the first place. Most of these approaches are do-it-yourself, but when your particular symptom could either potentially be helped by a prescription medication or warrants medical attention, I'll let you know. For the most part, these are things you can add to the treatment plan for your primary symptom set—then either potentially remove them once the symptom has resolved (in the case of a urinary tract infection, for example), or continue utilizing them as part of your new normal (such as adapting your skin-care routine to accommodate drier skin).

Having this information in your back pocket gives you some agency over your experience, which is a beautiful thing. But before we proceed, a quick reminder: Be sure to discuss any supplements or other over-the-counter options you try with your clinician, as it's important they know what you are taking.

One-Off Symptoms from A to Z

The following are some common, sometimes weird, solo perimenopause symptoms and what you can do on your own to alleviate them.

Acne

If you're suffering from acne as part of your perimenopause package, first of all: Resist the urge to pick or pop. Perimenopausal acne likely stems from the rapid spikes and decreases of estrogen, which means you sometimes have a lot more testosterone than estrogen. Excess testosterone can trigger acne (and also produce chin hairs—and, unfortunately hair loss from your head). Many of the things that often accompany perimenopause can also play a contributing role, including stress, lack of sleep, and high glucose and insulin levels. Some medications may also trigger acne, including corticosteroids, lithium, thyroid hormones (particularly if the prescription is too weak or too strong), some antibiotics (such as tetracycline and streptomycin), and antiepileptic drugs.

What you can do:

- As much as you might be tempted to use abrasive skin-care products, such as heavy exfoliants, your skin is drier and a little less resilient than it used to be. Instead, use gentle cleansers containing salicylic acid, which unclogs pores; or benzoyl peroxide, which kills bacteria. Use oil-free, noncomedogenic (non-pore-clogging) moisturizers and makeup. Wash your face once or twice a day, and even though you may be dog tired at night, don't neglect removing your makeup.
- Speaking of makeup, if anything you're using is more than a year old, it's time to replace it, as it can harbor bacteria that can contribute to breakouts.
- Visit a dermatologist, who may prescribe topical antibiotics, topical retinoids that promote skin cell turnover and prevent clogged pores, drugs that counteract androgens (male hormones, including

testosterone), such as spironolactone or oral contraceptives, and treatments such as lasers or light systems that reduce oil production and lessen inflammation.

- Visit your primary care doctor to rule out conditions that may be contributing to acne, such as polycystic ovary syndrome, or the much rarer adrenal hyperplasia, and to discuss if any medications you're taking may be contributing.

Bloating and Gas

Perhaps you've experienced bloating in the days before your period—when progesterone drops in relation to estrogen (as it does at the end of your cycle), it cues your body to retain water, which can lead to bloating. In perimenopause, you are likely experiencing this ratio of high estrogen to low progesterone more frequently, and so you may be experiencing bloating more frequently than just those few days before your period. Perimenopause can also contribute to changes in the microbiome, and since your gut bacteria play an important role in digestion, if they are out of balance, you might experience more gas.

What you can do:

- Eat more gut-friendly foods, whether that's prebiotics (foods that contain insoluble fiber that good bacteria love to eat), such as avocado, asparagus, bananas, leeks, oats, and onions; or probiotics (foods that contain beneficial bacteria), such as kimchi, kombucha, sauerkraut, or yogurt.
- Make sure you're adequately hydrated, as dehydration may slow transit time through the digestive tract, which can contribute to gas.
- Take a short walk after most meals to encourage digestion.
- Notice if there are certain foods, such as beans, fried foods, or salty foods, that cause more bloating, and minimize those foods.
- Too much fiber without water can backfire and lead to constipation. Fiber is a bulking agent, not a motility agent, meaning it

increases stool volume but doesn't necessarily stimulate elimination, so don't overdo it, and make sure you're getting adequate hydration and movement—both of which enhance motility.

Breast Tenderness and Sore Nipples

The water retention that leads to bloating can also cause swollen, tender breasts. Since I know you're thinking it: Breast pain is rarely a sign of cancer.

What you can do:

- Consider switching to a well-fitting sports bra, as the mild compression can be comforting—a small study found that 85 percent of women with breast tenderness found relief when wearing a sports bra as their primary bra, compared to only 58 percent of women who experienced less discomfort when taking danazol (a prescription medication for fibrocystic breast disease)—and 42 percent of the women taking medication experienced unpleasant side effects.[1]
- Here, too, hydration can help, because if you're not getting enough water, your body will retain fluids in an attempt to stay lubricated, and that may lead to breast tenderness, or make it worse.
- Give your sore breasts some TLC. If you can stand it, apply cold packs to your aching breasts, as some women find this provides relief. Anything frozen will do, but bags of frozen peas are easy to mold to your breasts.
- Try an herbal supplement. Some women get relief from breast pain by taking evening primrose oil, which contains the essential fatty acid gamma-linolenic acid. While the research supporting this effect is mixed, a 2020 study found that women with mastalgia (i.e., breast pain) who took 1,300 mg of evening primrose oil twice a day experienced significant pain relief—far more than a control group that took acetaminophen did—after just six weeks. It's a low-risk proposition because evening primrose oil doesn't cause side effects.

- When nothing else helps, try an over-the-counter oral pain reliever, such as acetaminophen, ibuprofen, or naproxen. You could also try a topical pain relief cream.

Brittle Nails

Estrogen helps produce keratin—a protein that keeps the nails thick and strong. As estrogen declines, your nails become more brittle and are more likely to break, peel, or not grow. Estrogen also helps in collagen production—the most abundant protein in the body that keeps nails (as well as hair, skin, and connective tissues) resilient. In fact, collagen levels may decrease by 25 percent as estrogen drops.

Beyond hormones, deficiencies in B vitamins, calcium, fatty acids, and iron also contribute to brittle nails. Continuous use of gel nails, fake nails, and acetone nail polish remover also take a toll over time. Medical issues such as an underactive thyroid, Raynaud's syndrome (where your hands and feet experience an extreme reaction to cold due to reduced blood flow to the extremities), or fungal infection can also weaken nails.

What you can do:

- Just as with dry, itchy skin, hydration helps (see page 226 for more specific hydration tips).
- Moisturize, moisturize, moisturize. I am a big fan of nonscented hand creams (those fragrances are generally chemical in nature and can be drying), especially Eucerin, although shea butter and coconut oil are also rich emollients. Once or twice a week, apply a little extra hand cream before bed and then wear gloves to bed so that your hands and nails get an extra dose of hydration (and you don't get any on your sheets).
- Make sure you're getting plenty of biotin (vitamin B_6), which is key for strong nails and hair and is found in ample amounts in eggs, soybeans, nutritional yeast, and—if you like it—liver. If these foods aren't in your regular rotation and your nails are breaking, consider a biotin supplement—you need about 30 mcg per day total.

- Iron-rich foods (spinach, shellfish, beef, and beets); collagen (from bone broth, tough cuts of meat, or gelatin); and healthy fats (avocado, nuts, seeds, and olive oil) can also help repair brittle nails.
- Give your nails periodic breaks from polish, gel, and acrylics, and switch to an acetone-free nail polish remover.
- Be patient, as fingernails take several months to grow out, and toenails can take as long as a year and a half.

THE SCOOP ON COLLAGEN SUPPLEMENTS

Collagen is an abundant protein that is an integral component of skin, hair, nails, connective tissue, tendons, bones, and cartilage. It plays a role in tissue repair, the immune response, and communication between cells. Sadly, women typically lose up to 25 percent of their collagen within the first five years after menopause, contributing to wrinkles and a decline in joint health. While the loss of estrogen is likely a causative factor, so are smoking, excessive drinking, and sun damage.

Food sources of collagen include bone broth, chicken skin, tough cuts of meat, and gelatin—things many people don't eat regularly. For this reason, a collagen supplement may be helpful for combating some of that aging-related loss, although the benefits of supplementing are not as clear as they might seem.

There is a lot of content on social media praising collagen as a solution for nearly every age-related ailment under the sun. While the benefits of collagen supplementation hailed by influencers generally aren't backed by research, there is some data to suggest collagen does have a positive impact on skin health: a meta-analysis of nineteen studies with over eleven hundred participants (most of them women) found that supplementing with hydrolyzed collagen did improve skin elasticity, hydration, and the appearance of wrinkles.[2] A 2023 double-blind randomized control trial (considered the gold standard of study design) that followed healthy, middle-aged adults for as long as nine months found that people who took 10 grams of collagen per day reported that they could perform more activities of daily living, enjoyed better mental health scores, and experienced less chronic pain (although only those most regular exercisers experienced that reduction in pain).[3]

If you are seeking to support your joint and skin health, try taking 10 to 20 grams of collagen powder per day. As with anything, don't overdo it, or use it as an excuse to keep smoking, drinking excessively, or going out in the sun without protection. And as always, tell your physician about any supplements you are taking.

Burning Feet

Though we're not exactly sure why, estrogen shifts can affect the nervous system and lead to peripheral neuropathy—or nerve damage in the extremities that can cause zinging or burning sensations in the feet. The same water retention that may lead to breast tenderness can also cause your feet to swell, which applies pressure to nerves that may contribute to nerve damage over time.

Also, hot flashes and night sweats—which are the result of changes in the flow of blood through small blood vessels—can cause a spike in blood flow and heat to the feet, which can feel like burning. At night your body also directs blood flow to the extremities in order to reduce your core body temperature, which may exacerbate the burning sensations.

Other possible contributing factors include a deficiency in vitamin B_{12}, which helps to regulate the nervous system. B_{12} is primarily found in animal foods, so if you're a vegetarian or a vegan, you can easily become deficient, and that means you need supplementation. Levels of this vitamin also tend to decline as we age. Additionally, an underactive thyroid could affect blood flow to the feet.

What you can do:

- It may seem obvious, but soaking your feet in cool water can help quell the fire.
- Try a vitamin B_{12} supplement if you aren't able to eat meat, eggs, milk, dairy, salmon, or nutritional yeast (all good sources of B_{12}) regularly.
- Try a topical pain reliever, such as capsaicin gel or benzocaine, to numb your feet.
- Talk with your doctor, who may prescribe medications such as gabapentin, pregabalin, duloxetine, or amitriptyline, which are used off-label to treat nerve pain.

Chin Hairs

No, you're not turning into a witch—hair growing in places you never had hair before can occur because your brain has been asking your ovaries for estrogen, but since your ovaries have very little estrogen left to give, the brain may be tapping your adrenal glands to compensate for the missing estrogen. The adrenal glands may then be producing cortisol, a stress hormone; and testosterone, the male sex hormone that can cause hair growth. While most women in perimenopause will experience a decrease in testosterone, 10 percent of women will find that their testosterone rises—and hairs in new places like your chin, as well as acne, can be the result.

What you can do:

I hate to say it, because this advice is repeated so frequently that it's almost a joke, but do what you can to reduce your stress so that your adrenal glands can take a break and produce less cortisol and testosterone. Prioritize the sleep hygiene we learned about in chapter 5. Be honest—are you staying up late? Blowing off exercise because you're so busy and then having a hard time getting to sleep at night? You don't have to completely rearrange your life, but any small changes you can make to lower your stress can help. Try doing ten minutes of yoga every morning or just before bed; try stretching while you watch a show at night; going for a walk or doing some other low-intensity exercise; and avoiding stressful situations with family or friends. For over-the-counter stress support, try:

- Ashwagandha is an adaptogenic herb (meaning, it helps your body respond to stress appropriately) used in Ayurvedic medicine that studies have found to be more effective at reducing stress and anxiety than placebo. Try 500 to 600 mg at bedtime for gentle relaxation.
- Magnesium glycinate, a bioavailable form of magnesium, is a mineral that is also a relaxant. Try taking 325 mg just before bed.

If chin hairs are really bothering you, you can also try laser hair removal, although it can be expensive, especially if you need multiple visits. There is no guarantee that this type of hair removal is permanent, no matter what the marketing materials say.

Clumsiness

Clumsiness can add insult to potential injury by making you feel like a hot mess. There are a few factors that may be combining to make you more prone to dropping or bumping into things, falling, or cutting yourself: The brain changes that declining estrogen and progesterone trigger may show up in impairment of your coordination, fine motor skills, and spatial ability. Meaning, you may be less aware of where you are in relation to the things around you, and less able to steer clear of things. On top of that, moisture levels in your inner ear change, and this can impair your balance. If your sleep is impaired and you're not feeling well-rested, that may also dull your reflexes and your coordination. If you're also experiencing symptoms like vertigo or dry eyes (that may make your vision a little blurry), this can further challenge your coordination.

What you can do:

- Regular exercise is always a good idea, but especially strength training—to help you maintain your stability—and anything that promotes body awareness and balance, such as yoga, tai chi, or Pilates.

- I know we all have so much on our plates, but if clumsiness is impacting your well-being, it may be a sign to move a little more slowly and stick to one thing at a time.
- See chapter 5 and review the list of sleep hygiene tips so that you get more rest.

Dry Eyes

Declining testosterone affects glands on your eyelids that produce the oil and tears that keep your eyes lubricated. Lowering estrogen levels impair hydration and lubrication throughout the body, including the eyes.

Aside from hormonal causes, research has also found a correlation between vitamin D deficiency and dry eyes, which can manifest as a gritty feeling, burning, itching, or redness.[4] Looking at screens for a large part of the day doesn't help, either.

What you can do:

- Staring at a screen can reduce the amount of times you blink by about half, making your eyes even drier. Switching your gaze to something nonelectronic is restful and promotes blinking. Set a timer for every twenty minutes to remind yourself to stop looking at your screen and look at something in the distance instead.
- If your room is very dry (such as in the winter when the heat is running), a humidifier will add ambient moisture to help prevent your eyes from drying out.
- Use a heated eye mask at the end of the day before bed to encourage the oil-producing glands in your eyelids to soften and produce more oil.
- Keep artificial tears in your desk drawer and your purse and apply them a few times a day, as needed.
- Take vitamin D supplements, which have been found to increase tear production and reduce the symptoms of dry eyes.[5]

- If these at-home attempts don't provide adequate relief, your doctor may prescribe cyclosporine to boost the production of tears and reduce inflammation, although it can take up to three months to notice the benefits. Another, faster-acting medication is lifitegrast ophthalmic solution, which also reduces inflammation and has been shown to produce noticeable benefits in only two weeks.

Dry, Itchy Skin

If your skin is feeling itchier, drier, or tighter than usual, you're not imagining it. Because estrogen helps us stay moisturized all over the body, when it declines the skin—your largest organ—definitely feels its absence.

You may notice dryness throughout the body, including the skin of your ears, both on the outside part of your ear as well as inside the ear canal. (I get so many questions about this on my social media—if you are feeling the need to scratch your ears like never before, you are by no means alone.)

This dryness may morph into skin sensitivity, where your clothes and jewelry feel uncomfortable in a way they never have before, or your skin is more easily irritated. If you're in the tactile sensitivity camp—some things just don't feel good on your skin—it may be because low estrogen can increase the release of histamine, a chemical most commonly associated with allergy symptoms. High histamine levels can not only cause redness, blotchiness, and sensitivity; they can also lead to histamine intolerance. That's when your cells become desensitized to histamine's messages, so your body tries to release increasing levels, resulting in a big allergic response.

What you can do:

- Take it easier on your skin—take warm, not hot showers, as water that is too hot will strip oils from your skin. Switch from deodorant soaps to something gentler, like liquid castile soap or goat's milk soap. Avoid products with synthetic fragrances, alcohol, and sulfates, as they can be drying.

- Lock in moisture by using richer creams, oils, or shea butter. (Again, avoiding those with synthetic fragrances.)
- Prioritize hydration. If you're not drinking enough water, it can affect your skin. Aim for at least sixty-four ounces of water per day. You can also get hydration through fruits and vegetables that have a high water content, such as melons, cucumbers, leafy greens, grapes, and carrots. Limit packaged foods, as they tend to be high in sodium, which is drying.
- Talk to your doctor about prescription antihistamines, such as Allegra or Zyrtec. While I don't recommend being on them for the long term because of their common side effects—drowsiness or amped energy, constipation, and dry eyes—they often help in the short term (and they are safe to use with hormone therapy).
- There are certain foods and beverages that are either high in histamine or promote its production. Try minimizing coffee, green tea, alcohol, fermented foods, processed foods, gluten, dairy, hard cheeses, strawberries, tropical fruits, and chocolate and see if it brings you relief. I understand that this list contains some frequently consumed, much-loved items. If you try cutting these things out for just a few days and notice a big difference in how you feel, you might be inspired to find a way to keep going.
- You can also try taking supplements of natural antihistamines, including vitamin C (small doses, such as 250 mg, taken three times throughout the day); L-glutamine (500 mg once a day); or quercetin (500 mg taken twice a day).
- While you've probably never thought about moisturizing your ears before, if your ears are itchy, be sure to apply moisturizer to your outer ears whenever you are moisturizing your face.
- If it's cold or very sunny outside, wear a hat that covers your ears, as both cold and sun tend to dry out skin.

- If your itching is in the ear canal, try applying a few drops of coconut or olive oil—just a little dab will do.
- If the itch is really bothersome, perhaps even making it difficult to sleep, try an over-the-counter anti-itch cream with a low percentage of hydrocortisone. If you feel that the itch is deep in the ear, make an appointment with your primary care doctor or an ear, nose, and throat (ENT) specialist.

Hair Changes (Curly to Straight and Vice Versa)

If it seems your hair no longer looks or behaves the way it did before you hit perimenopause, you're likely not imagining it. When estrogen starts trending downward, your hair follicles can get tighter, smaller, or a different shape, which then impacts the shape of the hairs that emerge from the follicles and the propensity of the hairs to curl. The hair itself can lose some strength and structural integrity, making it more vulnerable to breakage. Your scalp may start producing less sebum—the oil that moisturizes your scalp and hair—changing the pH levels of your scalp and making your hair prone to frizziness. (Frizz is the result of the cuticles on individual hairs opening up in search of moisture.) That change in pH can also cause your cuticles to become raised instead of smooth and contribute to your hair becoming coarse or wiry.

What you can do:

- Lower the temperature of the water you use to wash or rinse your hair. Just as hot water is drying for your skin, it also makes your scalp and hair more parched.
- Whether or not you're using shampoo, whenever you wet your hair, make sure to massage your scalp to promote circulation (delivering nutrients) and physically encourage old skin cells to move along so that they don't clog sebum-secreting glands or follicles.
- Add in a weekly pre-shampoo hair mask to up moisture levels in your hair and prevent frizz.

- A different hair texture or curl pattern likely requires different care—experiment with different shampoos, hair products, and styling routines. In general, the less heat you use on your hair (from blow-dryers, straighteners, or curling irons), the healthier your hair will be. A heat protectant is also helpful (and something I use daily as well).

Hair Loss

This is another unfortunate symptom of perimenopause. All the ways that hormonal shifts contribute to changes in your hair's texture can also lead to thinning hair—known as female pattern hair loss (FPHL). The loss of estrogen can also contribute to bald spots, thanks to hair shedding that outpaces hair regrowth, otherwise known as telogen effluvium. If you are experiencing higher androgen (male hormones, such as testosterone) levels in relation to estrogen as well, this also may promote thinning hair and balding.

What you can do:

- Treat your hair more gently. Avoid tight ponytails, vigorous brushing, color treatments, and high-heat styling, as they can all contribute to hair loss or breakage. Your hair is most vulnerable when it's wet, so blot hair dry instead of rubbing it with a towel. Let it air-dry as much as possible and use a moderate setting when you use a blow-dryer. You can also try sleeping in either a silk-lined sleeping cap or using a silk pillowcase to produce less friction on your hair as you move in your sleep and—theoretically, at least—less breakage.
- Many nutrients contribute to hair growth, including protein, B vitamins—particularly biotin (vitamin B_7); folate (vitamin B_9); and vitamin B_{12}—vitamin A, vitamin C, zinc, iron, magnesium, copper, and calcium. Make sure you're eating ample protein at every meal, and consider taking either a supplement formulated

for hair growth (check the ingredient list for these nutrients) or a multivitamin.

- For over-the-counter medication, try minoxidil (known as Rogaine) to stem hair loss and thinning on the top of your scalp. Sold as either an aerosol or a foam, you need to apply it every day and wait at least four months to assess if it's working.

- The yoga practice called balayam (which roughly translates to "hair exercise") is generally a form of moving meditation and is said to stimulate hair growth naturally. To practice, place your palms together with your fingers pointing up, curl your fingers into loose fists, and then firmly rub your nails across each other for five to ten minutes once or twice a day. There's no science to support its effectiveness, but the nerves in your fingertips are connected to the nerves in your scalp, and the practice is said to revive dormant hair follicles and improve blood flow to the scalp and follicles.

- Be patient. Hair regrows very slowly. With almost every method, it can take four, six, or even up to twelve months to see results.

- Consult with a doctor or dermatologist regarding other interventions. You may be a candidate for certain medications, such as the diuretic spironolactone (Aldactone, which has antiandrogenic effects); or finasteride (Propecia, which also counters androgens). As a bonus, these medications may also help with acne and unwanted facial hair, as those conditions can be triggered by excess androgens. In addition, there are is some evidence that noninvasive, unpainful laser treatments, known as red light therapy or cold laser therapy, are effective at increasing hair growth.[6] It's always a good idea to discuss whether your hair loss might be a side effect of any medications you're currently taking with your clinician.

- Although it's not FDA-approved for this usage, oral estrogen has some limited evidence to suggest that it is helpful in combating hair loss.[7]

Migraines

Fluctuating estrogen levels can contribute to migraines—in part due to the relationship between estrogen and serotonin—which means that some women experience an uptick in migraines during this transition. Lack of sleep is also a possible migraine trigger, along with weather changes, stress, certain foods, and even some smells (perfumes can be a huge trigger).

The good news is that migraines tend to lessen or even resolve post-menopause (unless you experience surgical menopause, which tends to worsen migraines). The bad news is that, depending on where you are in your transition, it could be several years before that relief happens.

What you can do:

• Try a complementary approach. I've had patients report that acupuncture has helped them reduce migraine intensity and frequency. Biofeedback—a modality that helps you objectively assess how you are responding to stress and consciously relax—has also been shown to be effective at treating migraines.[8]

• Prioritize your sleep. Review the sleep hygiene tips in chapter 4 to help you get more rest.

• Cognitive behavioral therapy (CBT) has also been shown to reduce migraine frequency and intensity.[9]

• Talk to your doctor about prescription medications, including triptans (which impede pain signals in the brain and can reduce nausea if that is part of your migraine experience); calcitonin gene-related peptide agonists (known as gepants, a newly developed class of drugs used to treat migraines); and drugs that influence serotonin levels, such as escitalopram and venlafaxine (antidepressants, although taken in lower doses when used for migraines). Supplemental estrogen or oral contraceptives may also be helpful—although not FDA-approved for this use, my patients report that stabilizing their hormone levels helps lessen migraine frequency. Although for some women, HT intensifies migraines.

Nausea

Just as changing hormones in pregnancy often trigger nausea, that can happen in perimenopause, too. Feeling sick to your stomach can also be a plus-one to hot flashes, dizziness, anxiety, and heart palpitations. Stress and fatigue—both of which can spike in perimenopause—also play a supporting role.

What you can do:

- Stay hydrated, as even mild dehydration can make nausea worse. Try to sip water throughout the day rather than downing a whole glass at once to avoid having a lot of liquid in your stomach, which could amp up queasiness.
- Acupuncture can alleviate nausea, as can acupressure, which is very similar to acupuncture but the practitioner presses on specific body points with their fingertips instead of using needles. Sea-Bands are acupressure wristbands that allow you to give yourself anti-nausea acupressure for as long as you have them on, and are available online and at many pharmacies.
- For an herbal approach, try ginger or chamomile. Ginger has long been hailed for its anti-nausea properties. You can take ginger as tea, lozenges, or candy. Chamomile tea, known for its soothing properties; and peppermint tea, a reliable stomach soother, also may help. Keep some of these options in your purse or desk drawer to have on hand wherever nausea strikes.
- Vitamin B_6, also known as pyridoxine, can help quell nausea, and has been found to be as effective as ginger in relieving nausea and vomiting in pregnant women.[10] Try 50 mg up to two times a day with meals if needed.
- Eat small meals throughout the day to avoid drops in blood sugar that may aggravate nausea, and try following a blander diet (no spicy, fatty, or sugary foods) until the nausea recedes.

Smell Sensitivity

Some women either become sensitive to smells that previously didn't bother them—such as the smell of coffee, or a perfume they used to love—or they experience what's known as phantom smells, where they smell something that isn't there, like body odors, smoke, or gasoline. We don't know exactly why this happens, but it may have to do with a general drying out of nasal tissues, which then impacts the olfactory system.

Rarely, changes in smell are a symptom of another condition, such as allergies or colds, COVID-19, hypo- or hyperthyroidism, Alzheimer's, or Parkinson's, so be sure to mention them to your clinician.

What you can do:

- If your sense of smell has diminished, try a zinc supplement, as zinc deficiency may contribute to a loss of smell.
- I've said it many times already in this chapter, but I'll say it again— stay hydrated. A humidifier is helpful for moisturizing those nasal tissues, especially if you live in a dry or cold climate.

Rage

As estrogen lessens, so does serotonin, which can diminish your emotional regulation—you experience a trigger, and you react (or overreact). The decline in estrogen also brings GABA, the calming neurotransmitter, down with it. Lessening progesterone plays a role, too, as progesterone is calming. So, it makes sense that when all of these are low you can lose touch with your sense of "chill." Combine that with perimenopause typically being a stressful time of life when you are also dealing with bothersome symptoms, like difficulty sleeping, and it's no wonder if you feel like you are spending too much of your time in a heated emotional state.

What you can do:

- Exercise is a great way to blow off stress and can also up the production of feel-good chemicals such as endorphins. It also makes you feel capable and strong. Use your piques of rage as a nudge to get moving instead of just stewing.

- Eat at regular intervals—every three to four hours—to avoid plunging blood sugar levels and that "hangry" feeling.

- Consider therapy. It's possible your rage is shining a light on some things you need to process. Cognitive behavioral therapy can help you objectively assess your thinking and restructure thought patterns that may be contributing to your frustration.

- Find places to safely vent. A regularly scheduled call or walk with a friend will give you both a space to get things off your chest and feel less alone in your feelings.

- Take a break and breathe. When the anger arises, if possible, remove yourself from the situation. Going into another room or to the bathroom can put a little buffer between you and your trigger and give your feelings a chance to settle before you react. Once you're there, imagine exhaling out your stress and irritation by breathing in for a count of three and breathing out for a count of six.

- Consider a gratitude journal or even make voice memos of what makes you feel happy and grateful. As soon as you are about to blow off steam, pop in your earbuds and listen to your own voice remind you of how amazing your life really is. (This is my latest hack for happiness—and something I talk more about in chapter 11.)

- Prioritize the things—or at least one thing—that makes you happy. Feeling overworked and underappreciated is enough to make you see red, even without hormonal fluctuations. Let your current anger spikes motivate you to commit to taking the time to do something just because you love doing it, whether that's gardening, writing, reading, dancing, meeting a friend for coffee or brunch, or something else that makes you feel good.

Tinnitus

Some perimenopausal women notice the onset of frequent or continuous ringing in one or both of their ears, although there is no recognizable external source of the noise. Known as tinnitus, it might sound like buzzing, pulsing, or throbbing that either starts or gets worse at some point during the perimenopausal transition.

Declining estrogen is likely at play, as it can dry out the inner ear canal and lead to decreased circulation to the ears, although science isn't exactly sure of the mechanism that connects tinnitus with perimenopause. Tinnitus also occurs in tandem with aging-related hearing loss, trauma to the inner ear from loud noises, an ear infection or a buildup of earwax, a head injury, temporomandibular joint (TMJ) disorders, diabetes, multiple sclerosis, some medications (including some diuretics, antibiotics, cancer drugs, antimalarial drugs, nonsteroidal anti-inflammatory medications, and antidepressants), Ménière's disease, or a circulatory issue.

What you can do:

- Bring the ringing in your ear or ears up with your clinician; they can refer you to an audiologist who will measure your hearing, or an ear, nose, and throat doctor to look for structural issues in the ear canal. They might also assess your cardiovascular health to rule out a circulatory issue, examine your ears to check for an ear infection, and discuss your medications to see if a switch might help relieve your tinnitus if it is disrupting your quality of life.
- Tinnitus can be alleviated by covering up the buzzing with other sounds, such as a white noise machine or music. Just be sure not to play music too loudly through your earbuds, as that could further damage your auditory system.
- While not FDA-approved to help tinnitus, some women find relief from tinnitus with hormone therapy.

Vertigo

Dizziness is a relatively common perimenopausal symptom, with 36 percent of women ages forty-five to sixty-five reporting that they experience it at least once a week.[11] Loss of estrogen sometimes triggers the estrogen receptors in your inner ears to go haywire, just like the receptors located in the brain do (which triggers hot flashes). Lowering estrogen changes the way your body regulates blood sugar and uses insulin, which could also be contributing factors.[12] Other symptoms, such as anxiety, fatigue, heart palpitations, high blood pressure, and hot flashes, also may trigger dizziness. It could also be the result of an infection called vestibulitis, which disrupts the fluid balance in your inner ear.

What you can do:

- First, give it some time. If it is vestibulitis (meaning there is an infectious or viral source), it should resolve itself in as little as a few days to a few weeks without any other intervention.
- In the meantime, stay hydrated, as dehydration can make you lightheaded.
- Instead of eating three meals a day, eat smaller, more frequent meals, in order to keep your blood sugar in a steadier state.
- Simple lifestyle changes, including being intentional when moving your head from side to side or moving slowly during vulnerable times like when you're getting out of bed, going from sitting to standing, or getting out of the tub or shower, help to avoid your blood pressure dropping suddenly, which contributes to lightheadedness or feeling faint. Choosing a fixed point to look at while making bigger movements (i.e., dressing or exercising) may also help.
- For an over-the-counter remedy, Dramamine might help allay dizziness and even nausea for longer car rides or flights.
- See your doctor to determine if there's an underlying medical condition. They can also refer you to vestibular rehab, which is similar to physical therapy in that it teaches you exercises that promote balance and stability that you can also do at home.

Urinary Incontinence

Perimenopause is often the first time women start leaking a little urine—maybe just when your bladder is full and you sneeze (known as "peezing") or laugh, or, maybe more frequently, when you run or jump.

This kind of urinary leakage is known as stress incontinence. Childbirth can take a toll on your pelvic floor muscles, as can a lot of sitting, poor posture, and just general aging, and when your pelvic floor weakens, it's harder for you to control the flow of or withhold urine. Excess weight gain is another stressor on the bladder. Losing estrogen only accelerates the aging of your urinary tissues, as it also takes a toll on the tissues of your urinary tract.

You may also experience urge incontinence, known as an overactive bladder, where you feel like you can't get to the bathroom fast enough. This is a result of your pelvic floor muscles contracting too often and can be exacerbated by alcohol, caffeine, a urinary tract infection, and constipation (where the buildup of stool will apply pressure to the bladder). Some medications for hypertension and some antidepressants can also be the culprits.

In either scenario, the fear of wetting your pants can make you avoid certain activities, like running, going to see a funny movie, or being in nature (and being far from a bathroom), but it is possible to alleviate the situation.

What you can do:

- Find and tone your pelvic floor muscles. I'm sure you've heard of Kegels, but they're not easy to do correctly (many women will engage their abs, glutes, or thighs instead of their pelvic floor). To find the correct muscles, the next time you are using the bathroom, try to stop the flow of urine. You may not be able to do it easily or completely, but that's okay—you're just seeking to identify which muscles you want to contract. Then, when you're not on the toilet, contract those muscles and those muscles alone for two to three seconds before releasing them. Work up to doing three sets of ten to fifteen contractions a day.
- Cut down on alcohol and caffeine, as they are both diuretics and can irritate the bladder.
- Drink plenty of water instead. Although many women will try to restrict fluid intake to minimize the need to urinate, that will just

reduce your bladder's capacity and promote constipation. Also, keeping the urine diluted is important for preventing urinary tract infections (which only increase the urge to urinate).

- Empty your bladder when it's full—not before. Some women will aim to use the bathroom as soon as they feel the urge, but that actually weakens the bladder muscles and can worsen the problem.
- Take steps to alleviate constipation. Drinking more water will help, as will taking walks, eating fermented foods or taking probiotics, and eating more fiber. This will help remove pressure from your bladder so you don't have to strain in order to have a bowel movement, which can weaken your pelvic floor muscles.
- Keep a change of underwear with you instead of relying on pads or panty liners to stay dry, as they trap bacteria that can lead to vaginal infection. (Remember, the purpose of underwear is to protect your pants—you don't need to protect your underwear, especially at the cost of irritating the sensitive labia with wearing pads your whole life!)
- If these measures don't help, talk to your clinician, who may refer you to a pelvic floor physical therapist, a urogynecologist, or biofeedback practitioners. Administering Botox to the bladder can be a helpful treatment for urge incontinence.
- Do the right exercises: You may want to avoid high-impact exercise (jumping rope/running/heavy lifting) and sit-ups, all of which can put pressure on the pelvic floor muscles.

Urinary Tract Infections

When there is plenty of estrogen on hand (meaning, when you are premenopausal), it helps to maintain an acidic pH in the vagina, making it an inhospitable place for infection-causing bacteria. As estrogen lowers, the pH elevates and becomes more basic, opening the door for bacteria to make themselves at home. In addition, declining estrogen also causes the tissues of the vagina and urinary tract to become thinner and more fragile, and thus more susceptible to infection.

What you can do:

- Vaginal moisturizers help to hydrate the tissue and create a thicker barrier between the outside world and the inside of the bladder. Look for products that contain moisturizers such as hyaluronic acid and vitamin E, and ones that don't include parabens, which are a class of preservatives believed to disrupt the function of estrogen (you don't need any additional disruption in this regard!).
- Stay hydrated, which will help you urinate more frequently and wash away bacteria. And go to the bathroom when you first notice that your bladder is full. Even though you may want to wait as long as you can because urinating may hurt, going too long can allow bacteria to build up. On the flip side, going too frequently (before your bladder is truly full) can contribute to an overactive bladder. You should also be sure to urinate after intercourse, which may help with UTI prevention by eliminating bacteria that may have built up around the urethra during sex. It works for some women, but not for others.
- Take care to wipe from front to back when using the bathroom, which reduces the chances of bacteria entering the urethra.
- If you are getting UTIs frequently, drink unsweetened cranberry juice or take cranberry supplements regularly, as they can help prevent bacteria from taking up residence on the wall of your bladder.
- If the infection persists or the symptoms are bothersome, make an appointment with your doctor or visit urgent care, who can confirm whether or not you have an infection and prescribe antibiotics if you do.
- Vaginal estrogen, which is safe for all women, is the most effective form of treatment for recurrent urinary tract infections. Even the American Urological Association (AUA) recommends it as the first-line treatment for recurrent UTIs. Urinary tract infections can cause severe life-threatening issues if the infection gets into the bloodstream, so it is not a stretch to say that vaginal estrogen saves women's lives!

- If you experience chills, fever, or pain in your back or side, this could be an indication that the infection has traveled to either your kidneys or your bloodstream (a life-threatening situation called urosepsis). Contact your health-care provider or visit urgent care right away.

Vaginal Dryness/Painful Sex

The vagina has the highest density of estrogen and even androgen receptors in the body, and as these hormones lessen, the vaginal tissues undergo significant changes—chief among them is a lack of moisture as our natural production of lubrication slows. The most obvious occasion when you may notice this lack of moisture is during sex—and perhaps even pain during sex due to the lack of elasticity in your tissues and a lack of lubrication; but it can also be felt when you are wiping after using the bathroom or while wearing tighter pants.

What you can do:

- If you haven't started to use lubrication when you have sex, now is the time. There is no shame in using or needing lube. Not only does lube make sex more comfortable, but it also increases the likelihood that you will have an orgasm. Some lubes also increase blood flow to your tissues, which helps with feeling and staying aroused. If you're using condoms for birth control, be sure to choose a water-based lube, as the oil-based kind can promote the risk of breakage (the package should clearly state which kind of lube it is). If not using condoms, I recommend oil-based, as it does last longer. In all instances, look for lubes with clean ingredients, such as Good Clean Love or Überlube. If you don't want to purchase anything special, coconut oil and olive oil also work well (remember not to use them with a condom, though).
- Just as it works to help prevent urinary tract infections, vaginal moisturizer can help to hydrate the tissue to keep it thicker, more elastic, and more resilient. Look for clean products with hyaluronic acid or vitamin E, and use it regularly.

- At the risk of sounding like a broken record—stay hydrated. That means at least eight glasses of water throughout the day, as well as eating plenty of high-water-content fruits and vegetables.
- Avoid using harsh soaps or bodywashes, as they are likely to contain alcohol, which is drying.
- And not surprisingly, my number one suggestion is topical vaginal estrogen. It is FDA-approved to reverse and prevent the genitourinary symptoms of menopause, one of which is vaginal dryness. It works wonders for vaginal dryness, and because it is local—and therefore does not enter the bloodstream and won't travel throughout the body—it is safe for everyone, even cancer survivors. It does require a prescription, however, so you'll have to discuss it with your clinician.

Yeast Infections

You can thank thinning vaginal tissue and changing vaginal pH levels for creating an environment where yeast can easily overgrow and cause telltale symptoms such as itching, redness, a thick white discharge, and pain while urinating or during sex. The way estrogen helps maintain a healthy vaginal pH is by promoting the growth of the friendly bacteria lactobacilli, which produce lactic acid. When estrogen levels drop and vaginal pH increases, it can lead to harmful microorganisms like Candida (the scientific name for yeast) overgrowing. That doesn't mean you're doomed to get recurring yeast infections throughout perimenopause. Sometimes it's just during times of hormonal change, which could be caused by changing birth control pills, or even adding vaginal estrogen, when Candida is given an opening—but when your hormones restabilize, your susceptibility will lessen. Even if you've had multiple yeast infections before, don't self-diagnose, as some sexually transmitted diseases produce similar symptoms. If you suspect that you have a yeast infection, talk to your clinician.

What you can do:

- Boost your immune system with vitamin C. Prime your defenses to fight off Candida by getting plenty of vitamin C from citrus fruits, berries, peppers, kiwi, broccoli, brussels sprouts, and grape-fruit juice. If you're not eating a lot of fresh foods, consider a vita-min C supplement of 500 to 1,000 mg per day. More vitamin C is not necessarily better—taking too much can cause stomach upset and diarrhea.

- Let your vagina breathe. Candida thrives in a warm, moist envi-ronment. Keep things cool by wearing breathable underwear with a cotton crotch during the day and taking your underwear off when you sleep at night (try sleep shorts or a long nightgown if sleeping au naturel isn't your thing).

- Tea tree oil is a natural antifungal. Mix a few drops with a tea-spoon of coconut oil (don't use it undiluted, as it could burn your tissues) and apply it before bed, sleeping in a long nightgown so it doesn't get on your sheets.

- Up your intake of fermented foods, such as yogurt, sauerkraut, kimchi, or kombucha, as the friendly bacteria can limit the rise of Candida.

- Stop wearing panty liners, which act as breeding grounds for infections. If you are leaking urine on a regular basis, try wicking underwear such as Dear Kate or Knix, and see a urologist or uro-gynecologist so you can ditch the liners and pads.

- If the infection is persistent or prolonged, then consider talking to your doctor. Commonly prescribed medications include Diflucan, and the new medication Brexafemme, which works by blocking essential proteins that yeast needs to survive.

Perimenopause is a variable physiological process—your approach to it should be flexible, too. I hope that this list of symptoms and potential remedies helps you find relief and reminds you that you always have options. As you continue along your menopausal transition, you can always refer back to these pages and decide how you want to adjust your care plan to accommodate either new symptoms that crop up or previ-ously bothersome symptoms that have gotten better or faded away.

While it's important to consult with your clinician about each of your symptoms and keep them apprised of any additional strategies you want to implement, ultimately, you hold the power to decide how you'll support your well-being and quality of life. By staying attuned to your symptoms, doing your research with trained experts (as you're doing by reading this book), and partnering with a menopause-savvy doctor, you have all the ingredients you need to enter the postmenopausal portion of your life feeling your best.

CHAPTER 11

Navigating the Transition with Confidence

Although this book is coming to an end, your transition will likely continue for another year or two (or several). I hope that *The Perimenopause Survival Guide* will remain a tool you continually refer back to as your experience unfolds and your body adapts to your new hormonal reality. As you continue to identify any new symptoms that may arise and work to address them—both in partnership with your clinician and on your own—you will not only be making yourself feel better in the here and now, but you will also be making the transition to your postmenopausal decades much smoother.

Tracking and taking steps to address your symptoms—whether through lifestyle changes or hormone therapy—also bolsters your health in numerous important ways:

- **You learn what works, and what doesn't work, for your body—** whether that's a treatment such as an estradiol patch or an IUD, or a specific supplement, a support group, or a sleep routine. You're continuing to build your knowledge about how to provide your body what it needs to thrive. And on the flip side, you might also now have a better understanding of what does not work, or what causes unpleasant or unnecessary side effects. The more you know about your body, the better.

- **Your mood improves.** Knowing that you have a plan and an array of tools to help you navigate your hormonal transition is much more empowering and comforting than feeling hopeless. More specifically, when it comes to mental health we know perimenopause can contribute to mood disruptions that can be misdiagnosed and mistreated as anxiety or depression, when in fact the mood changes are hormonally mediated. If you try an antidepressant, therapy, or both, but your depression or anxiety doesn't get better (because it is hormone-related), you may feel defeated, like there's no hope. But if you try hormone therapy and your mood improves, you know that you're addressing the cause and not just managing symptoms.

- **You lower your risk of chronic illness.** The steps you take to address your perimenopausal symptoms will contribute to better health later on. Getting more sleep, more movement, eating better, reducing your alcohol intake, and keeping up with your regular screenings (I'll talk more about this in just a moment) are each important preventive measures. Adding in hormone therapy—if it makes sense for you—may offer additional protection: Analysis of data collected from the Women's Health Initiative study shows that women who take hormone therapy within ten years of menopause tend to live 3.2 years longer, have less heart disease, and have a lower risk of developing diabetes and dementia or dying for any reason. In addition, their bones are stronger and their quality of life is higher.[1] While hormone therapy is not FDA-approved to treat or prevent chronic illnesses, plenty of data exists to show that women stay healthier and experience improvements in their self-rated quality of life. Getting started in perimenopause can give you a nudge in the right direction.

- **You may find relief for something seemingly unrelated.** Many of my patients discover that hormone therapy can be one stone that takes care of multiple birds. For example, Julie was experiencing body-wide joint aches and pains. To address this concern, she had an appointment at a top medical clinic to be tested for autoimmune joint diseases. In the meantime, she tried hormone therapy for her night sweats and poor sleep, and, surprisingly, her joint pain went away, suggesting that her dropping hormone levels were the cause of her pain. Julie was thrilled, and she canceled the trip to the faraway clinic. I've had other patients who were convinced they must have an autoimmune condition like fibromyalgia or chronic fatigue syndrome because of how tired they felt, but their sleep improved so dramatically on hormone therapy that they no longer felt like they had a mystery ailment.

- **You tend to enjoy better sexual satisfaction and sexual health.** If you want it to be, sex can be an integral part of your health and your life that boosts mood, sleep, and a feeling of intimacy with your partner—not to mention being a big source of pleasure. Of course, perimenopause does a number on vaginal health and libido. Taking either systemic or local vaginal estrogen (or both) to keep your vaginal tissues lubricated and strong helps to ward off vaginal dryness, pain during sex, urinary tract infections, and promote more pleasurable orgasms and sexual intimacy overall.

- **You build your self-care muscles.** Tuning in to your body and seeking to alleviate your symptoms now will help to establish a pattern of staying on top of your health going forward. Nearly every condition or disease is easier to treat when it's caught early. Flexing your self-care muscles will help you stay ahead of any potential medical issues. It will also better equip you to protect your quality of life and extend your healthspan—the number of years you stay well. Currently, the average person spends the last thirteen years of their life with some form of condition or disease.[2] I like to call this building generational health. While those years may seem a long way off, I bet you'd like to keep doing the things you currently enjoy when you're in your sixties, seventies, and eighties, whether that's skiing, biking, cooking, shopping, climbing stairs, or using fine motor skills for things like typing and painting. If you don't take care of yourself now, there is no magic pill coming for you in your later years.

Not only is there no medal for enduring unpleasant symptoms at any point in your life, letting symptoms go untreated can have serious and severe health consequences. If you're accustomed to acknowledging and tracking your symptoms because of your perimenopause experience, you'll help yourself stay in prevention mode and avoid treatment mode.

Paving the Way for Better Financial Health

There is a lot of data to show that women with untreated vasomotor symptoms and other menopausal symptoms retire early, meaning that as women reach the peak of their career, they find that they are simultaneously struggling with perimenopause and menopause, so much so that they leave the workforce. This affects everyone—employers, clients, colleagues, and of course families who may have to rely on a lower income. As you take steps to address your perimenopausal symptoms, it's also likely that the better you feel, the better your work prospects and financial health will tend to be.

Remember that Mayo Clinic survey I mentioned in the introduction? (If you don't, let's blame brain fog!) As a reminder, they found 13 percent of women had experienced a negative outcome at work because of those symptoms, and about one out of every ten women were missing days of work because of them. A British survey of four thousand women found that 10 percent of women ages forty-five to fifty-five had left a job because of their symptoms, 14 percent had reduced their hours, and 8 percent had not applied for a promotion.[3]

These stats have very real financial repercussions in the form of not only lost income, but also fewer Social Security benefits, and likely fewer contributions to retirement accounts. This is especially concerning considering that women live on average about six years longer than men, meaning women need more resources to cover our additional years of expenses (and to enjoy ourselves!). Addressing your symptoms will mean they don't have to take a toll on your livelihood.

My patient Jenna, forty-eight, was struggling with the "Dragging Yourself Through Life" symptom set. She experienced incapacitating fatigue and brain fog. At her job as an attorney, she was making mistakes that were impacting her performance and her self-esteem. While she was on a path to become a partner in the firm, she was scared that she wouldn't be able to handle the added responsibility and stress. Jenna had recently remarried, but she and her new husband weren't having sex much even though they were newlyweds, because she just didn't have the energy or the interest.

We started her on estradiol gel, but it was hard for her to remember to take it every day. Once we switched to a transdermal estradiol patch, she had fewer night sweats and started sleeping better, and as a result she felt like her cognitive function came back online. After a few months we added in progesterone, to protect her uterus and also to help even more with sleep, and we also added testosterone for her low libido.

Once she wasn't completely fatigued each day, Jenna made it a point to start taking a twenty-minute walk either before work or at lunch, and she signed up for a group strength training class with her sister on the weekends. As her energy and clarity returned, she stopped second-guessing her lawyering skills and went for that promotion to partner. Three years later, Jenna hasn't had a period in fourteen months—we celebrated her menopausal birthday at her last appointment, but honestly, it was a little anticlimactic because she has been feeling good for a while now. Hers is a true perimenopause success story!

Tending to Your Health from Here on Out

How your health pans out in the long term depends on the self-care and lifestyle habits you form today. Now is the time to really dial in the four pillars of health I outlined in chapter 9, "The Silent Symptoms." If you skipped over that chapter because you have a different primary collection of symptoms, you should go back and read it because it addresses things that every single person born with ovaries needs to do to protect their health and well-being in their post-reproductive years. In that chapter, you'll find strategies for getting good sleep now and into the future, nourishing yourself with the nutrients you need to stay resilient, tending to your mental health, and getting the movement that will help your heart, bones, muscles, and brain stay strong in the decades to come.

Getting more attuned to and proactive about your health now is how you maintain resilience and vitality for the next several decades (i.e., build generational health). The better care you take now, the less ground you'll have to make up later.

A key part of paving the way toward a longer healthspan is to get your care team in place and work with them to stay on top of your medical care, particularly your screenings.

Members of Your Care Team

Primary care physician

Menopause-certified doctor

Gynecologist

Dentist

As needed:

Therapist

Nutritionist

Fitness trainer

Physical therapist

ASSEMBLING YOUR CARE TEAM

A key part of building generational health is creating a care team you trust. You don't necessarily have to work with every type of specialist on this list, but they each can help you stay on top of both your own markers of health as well as the latest thinking and strategies for protecting your well-being.

- **A primary care physician/general practitioner/internist/ family medicine doctor,** who can keep an eye on the big picture of your health (including reviewing results and notes from your appointments with the other specialists on this list). They will likely be the one to give you an annual physical, order and review the results of your screenings, monitor your vital signs (such as blood pressure and cholesterol levels), and keep you on track with your age-appropriate immunizations.
- **A gynecologist,** who will order your mammograms and keep track of your Pap smears. They can also help you with birth control and monitor any irregular bleeding.
- **A menopause-certified doctor** to create and monitor your perimenopausal plan and really home in on treating your perimenopause symptoms. This could potentially also be your PCP or your gynecologist, although as of this writing there are still not many primary care physicians or even gynecologists who are adequately trained in menopause care.
- **A dentist** is important for everyone of all genders and identities, but especially for those of us who will go through perimenopause, because the drop in estrogen may lead to a corresponding decrease in gum health. Also, the bone density loss that perimenopause can usher in also extends to your jaw, which makes you more vulnerable to tooth loss.

- **A therapist.** Perimenopause is a stressful time, and declining hormones can take a toll on your mental health. Mood is such a key component of health, not to mention quality of life, so if you suspect yours is trending in a downward direction, you'll really want to address it quickly. If finding a therapist near you feels too hard, there are online therapy platforms, such as BetterHelp and Talkspace, that can make it easier to fit therapy into your schedule. There are also apps you can engage with at your own pace, such as Calm, Happify, Headspace, and MindShift CBT.
- **A personal trainer** or group strength training class will help you reap the benefits of building muscle. If you have budgetary or time constraints, there are many trainers who post strength workouts for women on YouTube.
- **A physical therapist** is great for helping to manage unresolved pelvic pain from birth, hip pain from carrying kids, or migraines or chronic pain from bad posture, and they are often covered by insurance.
- **A nutritionist or dietitian** can be incredibly helpful in figuring out how to truly nourish your body. If working one-on-one isn't in the cards for you for any reason, I recommend the psychology-based weight-loss app Noom to my patients. I also included two of my favorite books on diet and nutrition for perimenopause in "Appendix B: Resources" at the end of this book.

The Screenings You Need Going Forward

If you're like most women, perimenopause is the first time you'll have really interacted with the medical system outside of fertility treatments and childbirth, if you had children, or perhaps your yearly physical. Now that the seal is broken, it's time to keep that relationship going by partnering with your doctor to keep tabs on your health going forward, through both regular office visits and screening tests.

These are the appointments and screenings I recommend my patients get and how often. While different health organizations establish—and frequently update—guidelines on when women should have which screenings, you may need to have these done at different intervals based on your personal health history, family history, or current symptoms.

Most are covered by insurance as they are preventive care, although this may vary depending on your provider, your plan, and your age (if you are opting to get one of these screenings outside of the recommended age range).

Annual Physicals

An annual physical with your primary care physician is the perfect time to get a look at multiple factors of your health, both to assess your risk for certain diseases and conditions and to track your markers of health over time. At this appointment, your doctor should test the following:

- **Blood pressure,** which is a measure of the force your blood is applying to your arterial walls. There are two numbers in a blood pressure reading. The first reflects systolic pressure, which is the amount of pressure experienced while your heart is beating. The second quantifies diastolic pressure, which is the amount of pressure in the arteries between heartbeats. When overall blood pressure is high, which is defined as above 140 over 90 mm Hg more than once, this condition increases your risk of cardiovascular disease (the number one killer of women) as well as being a risk factor for cognitive decline (and a full two-thirds of dementia patients are women).[4] In women, blood pressure tends to rise around the time of menopause due to a combination of factors, including the loss of estrogen (which makes blood vessels less pliable), weight gain, or increased sensitivity to salt (which can happen after menopause).[5] After age forty-five, more women develop high blood pressure than men do.[6]

The official guidance from the American Heart Association is to have your blood pressure checked at least every two years, but most doctors will check it at every appointment. If you had gestational hypertension, preeclampsia, or eclampsia, I recommend having your blood pressure checked at least annually if not twice a year. Getting regular exercise, eating a healthy diet rich in vegetables and fiber and low in saturated fats, prioritizing sleep, reducing stress, quitting smoking, and limiting alcohol to one drink per day or less can help keep your blood pressure in a healthy range. Finally, white coat hypertension can rise in perimenopause as we are more prone to anxiety—meaning, your blood pressure jumps up at an appointment just due to the stress of being in a doctor's office or a hospital. If you think that this could be happening to you, I highly recommend keeping a blood pressure cuff at home and monitoring while you are comfortably in your own space.

- **Cholesterol levels,** which are also an indicator of the risk of heart disease and stroke. The menopausal transition is generally not kind to cholesterol—it is associated with an increase in total cholesterol, triglycerides, and low-density lipoprotein (LDL, aka the "bad" cholesterol), and a decrease in high-density lipoprotein (HDL, aka the "good" cholesterol).

The National Heart, Lung, and Blood Institute (NHLBI) recommends that women under age fifty-five have their cholesterol checked every five years, and women ages fifty-five to sixty-five every one to two years. So, it may be a little early yet to have your cholesterol levels checked regularly, which is done via a simple test known as a lipid panel that requires a blood draw at your doctor's office or a lab. However, if it's been a few years since you last had it checked, you may want to ask your doctor to test your levels now so that you can establish a baseline. I encourage my patients to do this yearly, because these recommendations are based on male physiology—which does not include plummeting hormones!

If your cholesterol is high, your doctor may prescribe statin medications to lower your levels. Non-medication approaches include the same approaches to lowering blood pressure, as well as swapping in fish for red meat as a source of protein and eating more spices—such as garlic, turmeric, ginger, black pepper, and cinnamon—as these can improve cholesterol levels when eaten regularly. Healthy levels are up to 200 mg/dL for total cholesterol; less than 100 mg/dL for LDL; and at least 50 mg/dL for HDL.

- **Blood sugar levels,** as measured by your fasting glucose levels (which reflect your blood sugar after not eating for at least eight hours) or your hemoglobin A1C (which gives you the average glucose level for the last three months), indicate whether you have prediabetes or diabetes. It's important to start checking these numbers, as your risk of diabetes increases after menopause. For glucose, anything less than 99 mg/dL is considered normal; 100–125 mg/dL is prediabetic; and 126 mg/dL or higher means you have diabetes. An A1C under 5.7 percent is normal; 5.7–6.4 percent is prediabetic, and 6.5 percent or higher is diabetic.

  Once you are forty-five, you should have your glucose levels tested annually. If you're not yet forty-five but are overweight or obese, had gestational diabetes, have a family history of diabetes, exercise less than three times per week, or have polycystic ovary syndrome, you'll also want to have your levels tested regularly.

  If your levels are high, in addition to tending to your four pillars of health, blood sugar levels become more of a focus. There are medications, such as metformin and semaglutides, that may also help.

- **Thyroid function** can be assessed with a blood test, known as a thyroid panel, that measures levels of different forms of thyroid hormones. Your thyroid gland runs multiple functions in your body, including metabolism, heart rate, and weight, and research shows that the risk of having an underactive thyroid rises significantly in late perimenopause.[7] While there isn't a consensus about when you should be screened for thyroid dysfunction, I recommend every woman age fifty and older be screened every year, or if you are younger than that but have symptoms of hypothyroidism, including fatigue, weight gain, dry skin, cold sensitivity, and constipation. If your results suggest your thyroid is struggling, your doctor can suggest treatment options.

Cancer Screenings

The risk of cancer increases with age across the board, although we have seen some disturbing trends in younger adults experiencing higher rates of cancer, too. Cancer is often much easier to treat the earlier you catch it, and luckily we do have effective screening methods for some of the most common forms.

- **Mammograms** screen for breast cancer by x-raying your breast tissue from two different angles while your breast is compressed between two plates. It's not comfortable, but a good technician can make it as quick and painless as possible. The American Cancer Society (ACS) and the American College of Obstetricians and Gynecologists (ACOG) recommend that women forty and over get a mammogram every year, while the United States Preventive Services Task Force (USPSTF) recommends you get one every two years based on your family history and shared decision-making with your clinician starting between the ages of forty and fifty.

   If you have what are known as dense breasts, which is more common the younger you are and affects about half of women, this can make mammograms harder to read (although it itself is *not* an independent risk factor for cancer). All this means is that your doctor is likely to order a second screening modality, such as an ultrasound, 3D tomosynthesis, or MRI, especially if you have a high risk of breast cancer due to genetic markers or due to a personal history of breast cancer or a strong family history. Because having dense breast tissue is so common in perimenopause, I let all my patients know that they should almost expect a secondary screening test and not to worry unless there is a diagnosis.

- **Pap smears and human papillomavirus (HPV) tests** use a swab of your cervical tissue (the Pap smear) to check for precancerous cells or the presence of HPV (the cause of cervical cancer) so that any suspicious or precancerous cells can be removed or treated before cancer starts. These tests can be performed at the same time in the doctor's office or clinic.

  The recommendations for these cervical cancer screenings are a little confusing, quite honestly. For women ages thirty to sixty-five, the USPSTF currently recommends a Pap test every three years; or a Pap test and an HPV test, done together, every five years; or an HPV test alone every five years—all of these recommendations are based on having previous Pap tests results that were consistently normal. If your Pap test reflects abnormal cells, your doctor will likely want you to get one every year, or put you on a schedule recommend by ASCCP (the American Society for Colposcopy and Cervical Pathology).

  It's important to know that when you are perimenopausal there is a higher likelihood that you will get an abnormal result, due to the general atrophying of vaginal and cervical tissues and the inflammation that can arise as a result of the loss of estrogen. The good news here is that the use of local or systemic estrogen tends to reverse vaginal atrophy—and those abnormal Pap results. Be sure to bring this up with your doctor if you wonder about getting a false positive result.

- **A colonoscopy or fecal occult blood test** are both screening methods for colorectal cancer, the third most common form of cancer in the US. The US Preventive Services Task Force recommends getting your first colon cancer screening at age forty-five—and earlier if you have a family history of colon cancer or polyps or irritable bowel disease. There are two primary methods of screening for colon cancer—direct visualization or stool-based tests.

The direct visualization methods include the colonoscopy, where you are anesthetized and a doctor uses a thin, flexible, lighted tube to look for polyps throughout the rectum and entire colon—and removes any growths during the procedure. There's also the flexible sigmoidoscopy, which uses a similar device to examine the rectum and the lower part of the colon; and computed tomography colonography (also known as a virtual colonoscopy) that uses X-rays and computer modeling to create images of the entire colon. If your results are normal, the guidelines call for repeating the colonoscopy every ten years, and a CT colonography or flexible sigmoidoscopy every five years. In general, the prep for these tests (which essentially requires you to take enough laxatives the day and night before the procedure to completely empty your bowels) is often worse than the procedure.

Less invasive are the stool-based tests, which analyze a stool sample to either look for blood in the stool or look for DNA changes that suggest cancer. These tests should be performed more frequently—every one to three years. The downside to these tests is that if there is any abnormality, you are recommended to schedule a colonoscopy (although there can be many false positives).

Bone Density Screening

There's no two ways about it—menopause can be brutal on your bones, especially in the one to two years after your menopausal birthday. Guidelines don't call for women to get a bone density test—a painless and quick X-ray called a dual-energy X-ray absorptiometry (DXA) scan—until age sixty-five unless you have a primary risk factor, including if you take certain medications (such as aromatase inhibitors, glucocorticoids, or gonadotropin-releasing hormone agonists), have a parent who fractured a hip, smoke, consume excessive alcohol, have a low body weight, have malabsorption issues, or have had bariatric surgery.

I think sixty-five is far too late, as by this time, you've likely lost a significant amount of bone—after all, 50 percent of postmenopausal women will develop osteoporosis.[8] I also consider menopause to be a primary risk factor for osteoporosis, since declining estrogen promotes the formation and function of osteoclasts—cells that break down bone—as I mentioned in the "Bones" section of chapter 1.

If you are in late perimenopause, you could discuss getting an early DXA scan. If your results show that you have osteopenia—the precursor to osteoporosis—it will help motivate you to stick to your strength training (which helps build bone); get more weight-bearing exercise (such as walking, which helps maintain bone); and get plenty of calcium and vitamin D (two nutrients instrumental in bone health).

This may feel like a lot of screenings. One tactic I've learned from my patients is to schedule as many appointments and screenings as possible during one week out of the year—get your mammogram, have your annual physical, and visit the lab to draw your blood within a few days of each other. While you're at it, take yourself out to lunch or get a nice coffee drink to make the experience somewhat pleasurable and then, you're mostly done for the next year. You're essentially time-blocking your appointments—and devoting time and energy to your health is definitely worth a reward. (This tactic also means you have fewer appointments popping up throughout the year.)

Embrace the Opportunities of This Time

I have sat across from enough women while they wept because they felt betrayed by their bodies. I know that perimenopause is not a gift. I'm not trying to bright-side you, or wave away what may be very real feelings of worry, fear, or hopelessness. You are entitled to all your feelings about perimenopause.

That being said, every challenge has opportunity baked into it. I hope that the strategies I've outlined in this book will help you feel stabilized, supported, and energized enough to consider the potential upside that this transition carries with it.

Some of this is borne out of necessity. If you don't take the time to observe your symptoms, find a perimenopause-savvy doctor, and try the tools and treatments that can alleviate those symptoms and shore up your long-term well-being, this can be the time when your health starts trending downward. Perimenopause is a wake-up call to put your oxygen mask on first.

As a physician, it's natural that my primary focus in helping women through perimenopause is health. I believe—thanks to my own research, education, and clinical experience—that it is well within our realm of agency to protect our health as we transition through perimenopause, and that by doing so, we also protect our health for the decades to come on the other side of this journey—menopause.

It does take time, effort, attention, and even some financial commitment to support your health over the long term—to stay on top of your screenings and doctor's appointments, to work movement into your life, to stick to a routine that allows you to sleep, and to choose healthy foods as often as you can. I see these efforts as investing in yourself, and that every small thing you do now will grow and pay dividends over time. Or, put a little differently, the more you take care of yourself now, the more you can enjoy your life now *and* later.

But there is another aspect of life that I wish more clinicians thought and talked about with their patients, and that is overall happiness and satisfaction. And here the news is very good for perimenopausal women. If you just read that and rolled your eyes because you've been feeling completely overwhelmed with how hard it has felt to keep your life together while also dealing with perimenopausal symptoms, I get it. Remember, I am right there with you. At the time of this writing, I am a mother to three kids under eight and am constantly running between business-building, playdates, sporting events, and the pressures of being a friend, wife, and daughter. I have many moments where I feel really down, wondering what the point of all this effort is. But here, too, I take comfort in the research, which both validates how I'm feeling now and gives me a grounded sense of optimism for what's to come.

There have been multiple large-scale studies involving American and European women that have found a predictable pattern to both happiness and overall life satisfaction, and it is U-shaped.[9] That means we tend to start our adult lives in our late teens and twenties fairly happy. Then this sense of emotional well-being starts to trend downward through the thirties before bottoming out in the mid- to late forties. Is it any wonder that this is the exact time of life when so many of us are in the throes of perimenopause? I think not.

But what comes next may surprise you—and that is that happiness starts to climb around the age of fifty. (Again—coincidence that the average age of menopause is fifty-one? No way.) And it continues to rise until people are in their mid-eighties, when it dips a little but still stays relatively high.

It makes sense if you are feeling like your happiness level is in the ditch now. *And* you have every reason to anticipate that it is temporary and on the verge of an upward trajectory.

Other positive trends to look forward to postmenopause that research suggests include feeling more patience and less stress (from the Australian study called the Women's Healthy Ageing Project);[10] feeling simultaneously more independent while also enjoying stronger relationships (from Britain's Jubilee Women study);[11] and experiencing a steady increase in self-confidence that eventually even exceeds men's (according to research published in the *Harvard Business Review*).[12]

There are also beneficial changes in the way our brains work that occur during the menopausal transition. In her book *The Menopause Brain*, neuroscientist Dr. Lisa Mosconi reports that the amygdala—the part of the brain that governs our emotional reactions to stressors— becomes less likely to be aroused by negative emotional inputs, and that postmenopausal women are more likely to respond from the prefrontal cortex, or the seat of logic and rational thinking, meaning we become less reactive.[13] Which likely helps explain why we feel more content and more self-confident.

While this research doesn't help with how you may be feeling at this particular time, it does offer hope for the not-so-distant future. In the meantime, I've always rolled my eyes when I've heard someone say you have to "choose happiness"—because who would ever choose *not* to be happy? But I've come to realize that expecting happiness to show up in the mail, or even to come as a result of putting a lot of effort into things you're proud of, whether that's your work, or your family, or both, is not going to lead to a sustained sense of contentment. It may bring spikes of dopamine (the neurochemical associated with reward and motivation), but those quickly fade, leaving you looking for the next hit. I've learned that a more lasting sense of happiness takes a sustained mindset shift and a strong internal sense of self.

One of the ways I seek to create this shift is to use my voice memo app to record self-affirmations (for example, "You're wonderful, you got this, you are prepared and fierce"); moments of gratitude (such as "I am so thankful for my mother picking up dinner tonight"); and to make note of positive things that happen and how they make me feel (great student and patient reviews are some of the most rewarding things; I read them into my app so that I can listen to them on my harder days). This process has helped me realize that many of the things I initially resist because they sound unpleasant—like getting out of bed in the morning to get a little movement or to do a meditation—actually have a significant impact on how I feel emotionally for the rest of the day.

I also find that seeing a cognitive behavioral therapist is extremely helpful in evaluating my thoughts and becoming better equipped to choose to pay attention to the thoughts that contribute to happiness rather than unhappiness. There is a little bit of rewiring of your brain that has to happen to help you make these choices again and again with less resistance, but right now, your brain is going through a reorganization anyway, so perhaps it's the perfect opportunity to make sure those changes are ones you want.

And really, this is one of the biggest opportunities that perimenopause presents—for you to start putting your needs and your happiness first. Of course, this may depend on your life circumstances—your kids and how old they are; if you're caring for aging parents or family members who need support. Not everyone is a caregiver, but if you are in the thick of parenting, or caring for an aging parent, or dealing with infertility treatments, or focused on building your career, perimenopause has a way of demanding that some of that focus goes back onto yourself. The payoff is that the more you tend to your needs now, the better positioned you'll be to sail smoothly into menopause and beyond.

Although you may not be feeling it quite yet, the day is coming where you'll be able to look back and see this as the start of a freer time in your life, a time to appreciate the wisdom you've earned and the self-advocacy and self-care muscles you've built.

Whenever your spirits need bolstering, remember: The best is yet to come.

Frequently Asked Questions

Because I get specific questions from women every day, some from my patients and some through my social accounts, I wanted to compile my answers to the most common ones here.

If HT isn't right for my risk profile, I can't tolerate it, or I just don't want to take it, what do I do? Am I doomed to have a bad perimenopausal experience?

No, you are definitely not doomed. There are three buckets of perimenopausal treatments: (1) lifestyle practices, including sleep hygiene, diet, exercise, supplements, behavioral changes; and complementary and alternative approaches (such as acupuncture and self-hypnosis); (2) non-hormonal medications, including two FDA-approved medications for low libido, two FDA-approved prescriptions for hot flashes, and one oral FDA-approved medication for the genitourinary symptoms of menopause; and (3) hormone therapy. This means you still have the first two buckets available to you. I cover sleep in chapter 4, diet in chapter 7, exercise in chapter 9, and supplements and other approaches throughout the book in the chapters that pertain to your primary symptom set.

The two FDA-approved medications for hot flashes are:

- Brisdelle, or paroxetine salt, 7.5 mg, which is the same medication used in the antidepressant Paxil but at a lower dose. It's effective because increased serotonin can decrease the frequency and severity of hot flashes—that's why many doctors have used antidepressants off-label for perimenopausal symptoms for years. Lower doses work better than higher doses.

- Veozah, or fezolinetant, binds to estrogen receptors in the hypothalamus, the part of the brain responsible for modulating body temperature. This medication helps to reduce core body temperature and helps with the heat intolerance that comes with hot flashes. With Veozah, it is recommended that you monitor your levels of liver enzymes, as it can rarely lead to elevated levels, which could increase the risk of liver abnormalities.

The two FDA-approved medications for low libido in women are (for more information about these, refer back to chapter 7):

- Addyi (flibanserin) is a daily oral medication for low libido that works by increasing dopamine and serotonin in small amounts in the brain. Increased dopamine can increase the motivation to pursue pleasure. It is currently FDA-approved for pre- and perimenopausal women, but not for menopause (although many menopausal women do use it off-label, successfully). As a bonus, my patients report that it also helps with mood and sleep.
- Vyleesi (bremelanotide) works on your brain's receptors for melanocortins, a family of hormones that play a role in sexual attraction and desire. It's an injection you self-administer as needed—I like to tell my patients to use it ninety minutes to two hours before date night, but its effects last several hours. Overall, this is a great option if you don't want to commit to a daily medication.

The FDA-approved nonhormonal medication for genitourinary symptoms is Osphena (ospemifene), a once-daily oral non-hormonal medication used to treat moderate to severe vaginal dryness and painful sexual intercourse caused by menopause. Osphena is a selective estrogen receptor modulator (SERM), meaning it works like estrogen in certain parts of the body (in this case, the vaginal tissues).

Remember, there is no one right path for perimenopause. We each have our own unique journey, and there is an approach that will work for you.

How long does it take for HT to work?

This really varies from woman to woman. On average, many patients will recognize some kind of body feedback within two weeks—you're likely to notice something has changed, for good (as in, you're sleeping better or experiencing fewer hot flashes) or for bad (such as you're experiencing breast tenderness or increased bleeding). For some women it takes as long as six weeks to notice a change. But for some women—and this happens so often in my practice that I don't think it can be the placebo effect—they feel differently within just a day or two. Once you have the feedback, if your results aren't to your liking, you can modify dosage, timing, and treatments until it is. This process will often take two to four months or more if you are very sensitive.

Will I gain weight on HT?

Most women ask me this question, which makes me wonder why: Is it that the messaging about estrogen is still negative, or do women feel like birth control caused weight gain and so, therefore, HT will, too? Interestingly, birth control pills are not linked to weight gain, but the time in a woman's life when she starts taking them is more likely to be the causal factor. Many women start taking birth control when they go off to college and their lifestyle changes dramatically. Weight gain around that time is more likely due to dietary habits and staying up late. However, many studies show that women who take HT gain less weight over time than women who don't take HT; and, importantly, they also have less diabetes, which suggests that HT plays a role in insulin resistance and overall metabolic health.[1]

The gist here is: Most women don't gain weight on HT. However, there are always outliers. If you try HT and do gain weight, it's important to share that with your clinician and reassess your treatment plan according to your priorities, symptoms, and medical history.

How does perimenopause affect fertility?

Fertility is dependent on both the quantity of eggs and the quality of eggs, and the further you are into perimenopause, the more each of these is likely to have declined. Also, with the lowering of estrogen, you may not be ovulating regularly, which makes it harder to know when you're most likely to become pregnant. That being said, until you've been without a period for a full year, it is still possible for you to get pregnant. I have seen plenty of patients who have been surprised by a later-in-life pregnancy.

While you can't increase either the quality or the quantity of eggs, a fertility clinic can administer hormones to encourage the ovaries to release more eggs if getting pregnant is your goal. These hormones will be at much higher doses than what is prescribed to treat symptoms of perimenopause. If you are trying to get pregnant, the tips in this book won't hurt. In fact, they may even help you ovulate more regularly. But they are not designed to help you get pregnant. If you are over forty and wish to get pregnant, I recommend booking a visit with a reproductive endocrinologist, because time is of the essence.

Is it safe to eat soy in perimenopause?

There is a persistent myth that because soy contains phytoestrogens it can increase the risk of breast cancer, but actually the opposite is true. Research has found that regular soy consumption *reduces* breast cancer risk.[2] The estrogenic effect of soy can actually be helpful in reducing perimenopausal symptoms because your estrogen levels are declining. Soy—whether in the form of edamame, tofu, unsweetened soy milk, or tempeh or miso (both of which are fermented, meaning they also provide probiotics)—is a great source of protein and beneficial phytochemicals. It's a good idea to opt for organic soy when you can, as pesticides are something we always want to reduce our consumption of.

If I have my ovaries removed, what kinds of symptoms can I expect?

If perimenopause has any evolutionary basis, it's to get your body used to gradually lower levels of hormones. If you are pre- or early perimenopausal and having your ovaries removed, it will immediately put you into surgical menopause, which can be quite a shock to the system because your hormones will drop instantaneously. While you may not have advance warning if you experience a medical emergency and need this kind of surgery, if at all possible, I recommend that all women who are planning to have both ovaries removed prepare in advance by scheduling an appointment with a menopause expert to discuss your hormone therapy options and have a plan ready to go immediately after surgery.

Perimenopausal or premenopausal women who have their ovaries removed tend to have worse symptoms, especially hot flashes, sleep disruptions, mood changes, and weight gain, compared to women who experience natural menopause. And the earlier in perimenopause you are, the bigger the shock to the system you are likely to experience.

If you are having a hysterectomy, or removal of the uterus, this technically does not include removal of the ovaries, but it is worth it to have a very clear discussion with your surgeon about what exactly they recommend you have removed. Because of the severity of menopausal symptoms that ovary removal can usher in, it should not be undertaken without a clear indication, such as risk for ovarian cancer, concerning cysts, or other medical conditions.

If you are experiencing surgical menopause, hormone therapy is the gold standard for reducing these symptoms if you are under the age of forty-five at the time of your ovarian removal and can use hormone replacement therapy, which many women can (that's why I suggest preparing ahead of time by seeing a menopause expert).

If you're already in menopause when you have your ovaries removed, you won't be thrust into surgical menopause in the same way, and your symptoms should not be much different than before you had the surgery.

If I didn't tolerate birth control pills, will I tolerate HT?

Oftentimes, yes. There are many differences in the formulation, dosage, and route of delivery between birth control and hormone therapy:

(1) Birth control uses synthetic hormones, such as ethanol estradiol and various synthetic progestins, the most common one being norethindrone, while most hormone therapy uses bioidentical, FDA-approved estradiol and Prometrium; (2) birth control dosages are upward of ten times higher than hormone therapy—they have to be higher in order to effectively stop ovulation (earlier, I explained if you're trying to have a baby, HT could help because it tends to stimulate ovarian tissue but does not suppress ovulation); (3) most of the time birth control is taken orally, while most hormone therapy estrogen is taken transdermally, which reduces the very small risk of developing a blood clot, and is often better tolerated in this route. And last, with birth control, the hormones are packaged together, and with hormone therapy, they are often administered separately, which is very helpful. If birth control didn't sit well with you, it was likely because of one of the hormones, but you couldn't tell which one (was it the estrogen or the progesterone?) or experiment with the dosage of the hormones separately. With perimenopausal HT, you can use the hormones separately, which I often do. I call this hormone stacking. The majority of women who have told me they didn't like birth control have not had a problem on HT.

When should I talk to my doctor about perimenopause?

When your symptoms are starting to affect your quality of life, especially if you've journaled and tracked your symptoms and tried some do-it-yourself approaches but your symptoms are still ruling your life more days than not.

Should I start HT if I don't have symptoms?

This one is tricky. There is no solid data to say that starting HT in perimenopause has long-term health benefits. It is still recommended—and FDA-approved—only to treat certain symptoms. However, you can—and should—talk to your doctor to ask questions and start to plan for the months and years ahead.

If I have a personal or family history of cancer, can I take HT?

There is no family history of disease that precludes you from taking HT, as there is no data suggesting that HT increases the risk of cancer or death from cancer. In fact, research shows that women on HT have a lower risk of dying from all cancers.[3]

If you are a cancer survivor, the decision regarding hormone therapy is very individualized. If your cancer was nonhormonal, you may still be a good candidate for HT, depending on your symptoms. If your cancer was hormone-related, the current guidelines state that HT is not recommended. However, you can still discuss your personal risk analysis with a knowledgeable clinician or menopause expert to gain more insight. There are always options to help the symptoms; you should never feel like you are left to suffer in silence.

How do I know when my HT dosage is right?

This is an easy answer: When you feel at minimum 70 percent better with little to no side effects.

How long can I take HT?

There is no end date for when you must come off hormone therapy, especially if you start it within ten years of menopause. Since I'm assuming that you are still in perimenopause because you are reading this book, you are in the clear. Sometimes women ask me if they should hold off on starting HT because they've heard they have only a ten-year window to be on it, but this is a misperception that stems, yet again, from the Women's Health Initiative Study. In the initial findings of that study, they documented that the risks of HT outweighed the benefits when women started oral synthetic hormones more than a decade after menopause. Because there is no time limit to the use of hormone therapy, if you are experiencing bothersome symptoms now, I don't suggest waiting, because reducing your suffering will likely give you a new lease on life!

Can you take vaginal estrogen and systemic estrogen?

Approximately 40 percent of women on systemic hormone therapy will also need local vaginal estrogen to treat their genitourinary symptoms (whether it's vaginal dryness, urinary incontinence, painful sex, frequent urinary tract infections, or vaginal atrophy). Vaginal and vulvar tissue is extremely dense in estrogen (and androgen) receptors and sometimes can use a little extra targeted help. And, because local vaginal estrogen does not travel systemically, this dose is not "adding" to the systemic dose, so there is no reason you cannot use both—and many of my patients do.

Can I use local vaginal estrogen if I have had a hormone-sensitive cancer?

There's no condition or treatment that prohibits you from using local vaginal estrogen—not breast cancer, chemotherapy, strokes, or heart attacks. The reason for this is again because local vaginal estrogen does not enter your bloodstream in any significant amount, therefore making local vaginal estrogen extremely safe. In fact, a study that followed women for eighteen years found that those who used local vaginal estrogen had no increased risks of chronic disease.[4] Other research has shown that women with a history of breast cancer using local vaginal estrogen did not have any recurrence of cancer related to the use of vaginal estrogen.[5] Unfortunately, despite this, the FDA requires that local vaginal estrogen carry the same scary-sounding black box warning that systemic oral and transdermal estrogen does, which is still based on the initial findings of the Women's Health Initiative, even though further analysis of the WHI data has shown that these risks are not the whole story.

How do I know I'm in perimenopause?

If you are over forty-five and reading this book, whether you have noticeable symptoms or not, odds are high that you are in perimenopause. (Or as a meme I saw recently said, if you watched *Saved by the Bell* after school, you are probably perimenopausal.) Even if you're younger but starting to notice some changes to your monthly cycles, you've likely started your menopausal transition.

As we've covered, there is no definitive lab test for perimenopause; if you're looking for an official diagnosis, you'll need to see a hormone-savvy clinician who will assess your symptoms and history and, yes, perhaps order lab tests to measure your hormone levels, even though the results of those tests are only helpful data points, not hard-and-fast criteria.

Sometimes hormone therapy can be a helpful diagnostic—if you try it and you feel better, your symptoms were hormonally mediated.

Should I get my hormone levels checked?

While lab tests won't confirm perimenopause, they can be helpful for establishing a baseline, easing your mind if you're a data junkie, or providing some insight into where you are in the perimenopausal process if you don't get periods (because you have an IUD, or have had an ablation). Although, if you're on any form of birth control (besides the IUD), your lab results have no bearing on whether you're in perimenopause because your hormone levels are affected by the medication. Any systemic hormonal contraception will give you low levels of follicle-stimulating hormone (FSH)—which may (potentially falsely) make it look like you are not very far into perimenopause, as FSH greater than 35 on more than one occasion is suggestive of menopause.

If your doctor does order labs, and you are not on systemic oral birth control, and your FSH comes back high, keep in mind that those results are capturing your level only on one day, not the trend. If you are going long stretches without a period, that could cause your FSH to rise temporarily—and you could still get a period next month (and therefore, not be in menopause). Trying to figure out what your FSH levels really mean is often a game you can play all day, but what's more important is actually treating your symptoms.

How do I know when to start HT?

When you've tried lifestyle changes to improve your health but you're not seeing improvements, it's time to seriously consider that your body is going through an unavoidable physiological process and could use some support. You can't out-yoga your declining hormone levels, so make that appointment and use the tools in chapter 1 to get set up for a successful visit with your clinician.

How long should I work with a menopause-certified clinician?

It is a long-term relationship. This clinician could be your primary care doctor or your gynecologist, or a physician who specializes in menopause care. In my practice, I like to see patients every two to three months until they tell me they feel at least 80 percent better and are happy with their treatment plan. After that, if you are perimenopausal, I like to check in every six months, as your hormonal reality is still shifting and you may need to make adjustments to your treatments a few times along the way. If you are postmenopausal, I recommend an annual appointment to continue to keep tabs on the effectiveness of your treatment plan and any changes in your health history that might require us to adjust our approach. At those annual visits, we discuss how you've been feeling, if you have any new health goals or developments, how you're tending to your four pillars of health, ensure you are up-to-date with your screening tests, and answer any questions you may have. With all the new social media attention menopause is getting, there are often lots of questions to unpack at each visit!

Resources

Finding a Clinician Trained in Perimenopause and Menopause

The Menopause Society Website's "Find a Menopause Practitioner" Section

This directory lists members of the Menopause Society as well as health-care professionals who have passed a competency exam and earned the Menopause Society Certified Practitioner credential and who are accepting new patients. Go to menopause.org, then click on "Find a Menopause Practitioner."

The Heather Hirsch Directory

This is a listing of everyone who has been certified through the Heather Hirsch Academy—my training course for clinicians (heatherhirschdirectory .com).

Finding a Medical Practice That Specializes in Treating Symptoms of Perimenopause and Menopause

Alloy

Provides online access to physicians who specialize in perimenopause and menopause care and who can prescribe hormone therapy and other medications to address your symptoms; available in all fifty states and Washington, DC (myalloy.com).

Evernow

A monthly membership that offers 24-7 access to trained providers via video or text and a personalized care plan that includes medication, self-guided programs, and more. The cost of medications is separate (evernow.com).

Heather Hirsch Collaborative

A private telemedicine practice staffed exclusively by clinicians trained by me. We are all guided by the principle of shared decision-making, and our services are available in nearly all fifty states. All of our patients are also invited to join a private Facebook group that provides the crucial ingredient to any challenging journey—community (heatherhirschmd.com/collaborative).

Midi Health

Offers virtual visits with clinicians who have completed Midi's training program who can prescribe medications when warranted and also advise on strategies you can implement on your own. Visits and some medications are covered by many different major insurance plans (joinmidi.com).

Finding a Therapist

Psychology Today

A great resource for finding a therapist near you—their listings provide photos and a message from each provider. You can also find out if they are accepting new patients, see their credentials, identify the insurance they accept, and retrieve their contact information. Go to Psychologytoday .com/us and click on "Find a Therapist."

Zencare

Another great resource that also offers a short video from each provider, their license information and educational background, what their peers have to say about their work, the hours they are available, and the modalities they use, as well as accepted insurance and contact information. Available only in California, Florida, Massachusetts, New York, Rhode Island, and Texas (zencare.co).

Sleep Support

Cognitive Behavioral Therapy for Insomnia (CBT-I)

There is an impressive body of research that establishes the effectiveness of cognitive behavioral therapy for insomnia in promoting healthy sleep. To find a provider trained in CBT-I, visit the Society of Behavioral Sleep Medicine (behavioralsleep.org); or the International Directory of CBT-I Providers maintained by the Perelman School of Medicine at the University of Pennsylvania (cbti.directory).

Evia App

The Menopause Society recommends self-hypnosis as an effective way to manage hot flashes, night sweats, and insomnia. The Evia app talks you through evidence-based hypnotherapy techniques, mental imagery, and guided relaxation to help you get more sleep (eviamenopause.com).

Bringing Down Costs of Prescription Medicine

- **GoodRx** is a website that allows you to comparison-shop the prices of prescription medications at different pharmacies in your area and provides coupon codes to add additional savings (goodrx.com).
- **Cost Plus Drugs** is an online discount pharmacy (founded by *Shark Tank* regular Mark Cuban) that fills prescriptions with generic medications that are generally at a substantially lower cost than what's available at your local pharmacy (costplusdrugs.com).
- **PhilRx** is another online discount pharmacy that works with your insurance provider to get you the lowest possible price (phil.us/patients).

If You Are a Clinician Who Would Like Training in Perimenopause and Menopause

Heather Hirsch Academy

I am so devoted to increasing the number of clinicians who are educated in women's hormonal care that I created my own course. If you are a prescribing health-care professional (including MDs, DOs, NPs, PAs, and pharmacists) and would like to be able to prescribe and manage hormone therapy with ease and confidence, visit heatherhirschacademy .com.

Websites and Apps for Perimenopausal Women

- **HelloPeri:** Founded by Maggie Ney, a naturopathic doctor and Menopause Society certified practitioner and marketing specialist Alisa Kasmer, HelloPeri offers virtual courses that educate and empower women to take control of their perimenopause experience (thehelloperi.com).
- **Perry:** This app provides access to a community of women who are also going through perimenopause (think a social media platform just for those in perimenopause), as well as personalized content and expert-led discussions (heyperry.com). They also have a podcast called *Perimenopause WTF?*
- **The Swell** is an online community and learning platform for the forty-plus crowd that also hosts in-person events—many focused on perimenopause and menopause (theswell.com).
- **Women Living Better,** founded by former consultant and biotech program manager Nina Coslov, is a website that both conducts research and communicates the latest research findings on the transition to menopause (womenlivingbetter.org).

Books

- *Estrogen Matters: Why Taking Hormones in Menopause Can Improve and Lengthen Women's Lives—Without Raising the Risk of Breast Cancer* (revised edition, 2024) by Avrum Bluming, MD, gives a deep dive into both the research-backed benefits of hormone therapy and the reasons why we feared it for so long.
- *The Galveston Diet: The Doctor-Developed, Patient-Proven Plan to Burn Fat and Tame Your Hormonal Symptoms* (2023) by Mary Claire Haver, MD, is a physician's guide to updating your nutrition in order to avoid the metabolic changes and weight gain so common in perimenopause and menopause, with a focus on quelling inflammation, incorporating intermittent fasting, and finding the right balance of protein, carbs, and fats to both lose belly fat and reduce your symptoms.
- *The Menopause Brain: New Science Empowers Women to Navigate the Pivotal Transition with Knowledge and Confidence* (2024) by Lisa Mosconi, PhD, is a neuroscientist's guide to the many ways the menopausal transition impacts the brain—and the many ways we can support our brains throughout. Mosconi also shares how menopause shapes our brain for the better. (Yes, you read that right!)
- *The Menopause Diet Plan: A Natural Guide to Managing Hormones, Health, and Happiness* (2020) by Hillary Wright, MEd, RN; and Elizabeth Ward, MS, RN, offers a commonsense, fad-free approach to eating in order to manage your weight and keep your heart, brain, and bones healthy while also reducing your risk of cancer and other chronic conditions.
- *Mind Over Menopause: Lose Weight, Love Your Body, and Embrace Life Over 50 with a Powerful New Mindset* (2023) by Pahla Bowers covers the mindset side of perimenopause and menopause—how to

process your feelings, rethink your attitude toward your body, let go of the idea that you need to diet, and embrace mindfulness so that you can navigate the transition on your own terms.

- *Reversing Alzheimer's: The New Toolkit to Improve Cognition and Protect Brain Health* (2024) by Heather Sandison, ND, shares the evidence-based protocol she uses with patients and memory care residents to either prevent or reverse cognitive decline. Because Alzheimer's is a disease that primarily affects women and the neurological changes that promote it tend to start around perimenopause—and at midlife you may be caring for a parent with dementia or Alzheimer's—I wanted to include this book, which makes a difficult, upsetting topic very clear, actionable, and even hopeful.

- *Unlock Your Menopause Type* (2023) by Heather Hirsch, MD, is my first book; it is meant to help you personalize your approach to treating your menopause symptoms. Admittedly, since you've read *The Perimenopause Survival Guide*, you're more likely to sail through menopause than to crash-land, but there are physiological differences between the two life stages and, thus, different treatment approaches. Gift it to an older friend or a loved one, and then borrow it once you hit your menopause birthday.

Medical Associations

American Academy of Sleep Medicine (AASM)

The only medical society devoted to sleep medicine. They produce a website geared toward providing patients with accurate, evidence-based information on sleep (sleepeducation.org).

American College of Obstetricians and Gynecologists (ACOG)

This professional medical association supports both obstetricians and gynecologists (through research and practice guidelines) and women throughout their lives (via education materials and initiatives to improve public health) (acog.org/womens-health).

American Council on Exercise (ACE)

This organization educates and certifies fitness professionals (should you decide to work with a trainer, it's a good idea to ask if they are ACE-certified). They have a comprehensive exercise library on their website that demonstrates proper form as well as numerous articles on healthy living on their blog (acefitness.org).

American Psychological Association (APA)

A private organization whose mission is to promote the advancement, communication, and application of psychological science in order to improve lives. Their website offers many timely articles geared toward patients on a range of psychological issues, from living through stressful times to mitigating anxiety (apa.org).

Endocrine Society

A global community of physicians and scientists devoted to advancing hormone research and improving quality of life and health outcomes for patients. Their website hosts a clearinghouse of evidence-based information on aspects of health that are hormonally related, including perimenopause (of course), as well as diabetes, osteoporosis, thyroid health, and obesity (endocrine.org).

International Society for the Study of Women's Sexual Health (ISSWSH)

A multidisciplinary, academic, and scientific organization devoted to providing vetted health information to patients and supporting the highest level of ethics in researching, teaching about, and practicing women's sexual health. Their site is informative for patients; it also contains a provider directory (isswsh.org).

The Menopause Society

An independent nonprofit that is a leading voice on evidence-based standards of care for perimenopausal and menopausal women. They certify practitioners, publish peer-reviewed research in their journal *Menopause*, and host events, such as their yearly conference, that provide continuing education. Their website has a lot of helpful information for patients, including the aforementioned directory of credentialed providers (menopause.org).

A Fill-in-the-Blank Script for Discussing Treatment Options with Your Doctor

Dr. _____,

For the last _____ months, I have felt the following symptoms:

1. _____

2. _____

3. _____

They are affecting my quality of life in the following ways:

1. _____

2. _____

3. _____

I have tried the following things to alleviate these symptoms [what you've tried and the results]:

1. _____

2. _____

3. _____

I would like to prioritize _____[symptom] first,

because _____[your reason].

And I would like to use shared decision-making to help me find the treatment that will be best for me based on my symptoms and the information I have already shared.

[If you are considering hormone therapy, add these remaining pieces.]

I have been working on _____,

_____, and _____ [lifestyle

changes], but I still feel that my body may benefit from hormone

therapy.

ACKNOWLEDGMENTS

First off, I want to acknowledge you, dear reader. In our connected world, honestly, one thirty-second TikTok video will likely reach more people than the typical book will. Thank you for taking the time to do a deeper dive into your health during this crucial time of life, and for trusting me to help you navigate that journey.

I want to thank my grandfather, my biggest hero. As an ob-gyn who believed in preventive care back in the 1950s, his example directly influenced my own path—although mine has been a little different than his.

I am so thankful for the guidance and expertise of my writing and publishing team, Kate Hanley; Nana K. Twumasi, Natalie Bautista, Jim Datz, Alexandra Hernandez, Alana Spendley, Deborah Wiseman, Tareth Mitch, and Pam Rehn at Hachette; and Jane von Mehren at Aevitas.

This book would not exist without my patients, who have given me endless inspiration and who have helped me see patterns that help women pick a starting point on their ever-winding journey.

I would not be the clinician I am today without my mentor Dr. Holly Thacker, professor of Obstetrics and Gynecology and the director of the Center for Specialized Women's Health at the Cleveland Clinic. Thank you for opening my eyes to the importance of women's midlife health, and igniting a desire and the resolve to challenge the status quo and work to improve quality of life and health outcomes for women who are transitioning through the end of their reproductive years.

A special thank-you to my friends and colleagues in the menopause community (or "the Menoposse" as we like to call it). You all motivate me and teach me on a daily basis, and I am so appreciative of all the work you do to increase awareness of these topics, and for putting yourself out there to be an example to me and others. I'm thrilled to say that there are more of you than I could possibly name and the list is growing every day. But I'd like to especially thank those of you who were early readers of this book: Kara Baskin, Dr. Avrum Bluming, Dr. Kelly Casperson, Tamsen Fadal, Dr. Rena Malik, and Dr. Rachel Rubin. Thank you to the amazing allied health-care professionals who are also working to bring education to women. And a special thanks to Lindsey Miller, ACSM-CPT, my best friend since childhood and personal trainer, who contributed the strength-training workouts available to you at heatherhirschmd.com/perimenopause as well.

It is the best feeling to be part of a team of such smart and passionate clinicians at the Collaborative by Heather Hirsch, MD, and the educators at the Heather Hirsch Academy. I would not be where I am without my ever-growing team, which includes the amazing Nihar Ganju, MD; Liz VanSkike; Betty Wang, MD; Alyssa Johnson; Rachel Buck; my social media manager, Katie Sottile; my executive assistant, Alene Morash; Donna Benner of Swoon Talent; my web designer, Ansley Fones; and all the amazing clinicians who work at my telemedicine practice, the Collaborative, by Heather Hirsch, MD.

Last, I could not have written this book without the support of my family, including my mother (who jokes she is my airport Uber driver); my husband, Blaze Hirsch; and my three amazing children.

NOTES

Introduction

1. J. A. Cauley, N. S. Wampler, J. M. Barnhart, L. Wu, M. Allison, Z. Chen, S. Hendrix, J. Robbins, R. D. Jackson, and Women's Health Initiative Observational Study, "Incidence of Fractures Compared to Cardiovascular Disease and Breast Cancer: The Women's Health Initiative Observational Study," *Osteoporosis International* 19, no. 12 (2008): 1717–23, https://doi.org/10.1007/s00198-008-0634-y.

2. Stephanie S. Faubion, Felicity Enders, Mary S. Hedges, Rajeev Chaudhry, Juliana M. Kling, Chrisandra L. Shufelt, Mariam Saadedine, Kristin Mara, Joan M. Griffin, and Ekta Kaptoor, "Impact of Menopause Symptoms on Women in the Workplace," *Mayo Clinic Proceedings*, 2023, https://doi.org/10.1016/j.mayocp.2023.02.025.

3. M. Geukes, M. P. van Aalst, S. J. Robroek, J. S. Laven, and H. Oosterhof, "The Impact of Menopause on Work Ability in Women with Severe Menopausal Symptoms," *Maturitas* 90 (2016): 3–8, https://doi.org/10.1016/j.maturitas.2016.05.001.

4. N. F. Woods, N. Coslov, and M. Richardson, "Anticipated Age of Perimenopausal Experiences, Stress, Satisfaction, and Health and Well-Being: Observations from the Women Living Better Survey," *Menopause* 30, no. 8 (2023): 807–16, https://doi.org/10.1097/GME.0000000000002206.

5. J. M. Kling, K. L. MacLaughlin, P. F. Schnatz, C. J. Crandall, L J. Skinner, C. A. Stuenkel, A. M. Kaunitz, D. L. Bitner, K. Mara, K. S. Fohmader Hilsaca, and S. S. Faubion, "Menopause Management Knowledge in Postgraduate Family Medicine, Internal Medicine, and Obstetrics and Gynecology Residents: A Cross-Sectional Survey," *Mayo Clinic Proceedings* 94, no. 2 (2019): 242–53, https://doi.org/10.1016/j.mayocp.2018.08.033.

Chapter 1

1. "Launch of White House Initiative on Women's Health Research," White House, November 17, 2023, https://www.whitehouse.gov/gpc/briefing-room/2023/11/17/launch-of-white-house-initiative-on-womens-health-research/.

2. "Key Statistics for Breast Cancer," American Cancer Society, retrieved February 12, 2024, from https://www.cancer.org/cancer/types/breast-cancer/about/how-common-is-breast-cancer.html.

3. F. Sultana, S. R. Davis, R. J. Bell, S. Taylor, and R. M. Islam, "Association Between Testosterone and Cognitive Performance in Postmenopausal Women: A Systematic Review of Observational Studies," *Climacteric* 26, no. 1 (2023): 5–14, https://doi.org/10.1080/13697137.2022.2139600.

4. Samar R. El Khoudary, Brooke Aggarwal, Theresa M. Beckie, Howard N. Hodis, Amber E. Johnson, Robert D. Langer, Marian C. Limacher, et al., "Menopause Transition and Cardiovascular Disease Risk: Implications for Timing of Early Prevention: A Scientific Statement from the American Heart Association," *Circulation* 142, no. 25 (2020): e506-e532, https://doi.org/10.1161/CIR.0000000000000912.

5. T. Saaresranta and O. Polo, "Hormones and Breathing," *Chest* 122, no. 6 (2002): 2165–82, https://doi.org/10.1378/chest.122.6.2165; C. Dimitropoulou, F. Drakopanagiotakis, and J. D. Catravas, "Estrogen as a New Therapeutic Target for Asthma and Chronic Obstructive Pulmonary Disease," *Drug News & Perspectives* 20, no. 4 (2007): 241–52, https://doi.org/10.1358/dnp.2007.20.4.1103523.

6. H. Pang, S. Chen, D. M. Klyne, et al., "Low Back Pain and Osteoarthritis Pain: A Perspective of Estrogen," *Bone Research* 11, no. 42 (2023), https://doi.org/10.1038/s41413-023-00280-x.

7. Vonda J. Wright, Jonathan D. Schwartzman, Rafael Itinoche, and Jocelyn Wittstein, "The Musculoskeletal Syndrome of Menopause," *Climacteric* (2024): 1–7, https://doi.org/10.1080/13697137.2024.2380363.

8. F. Mauvais-Jarvis, J. E. Manson, J. C. Stevenson, and V. A. Fonseca, "Menopausal Hormone Therapy and Type 2 Diabetes Prevention: Evidence, Mechanisms, and Clinical Implications," *Endocrine Reviews* 38, no. 3 (2017): 173–88, https://doi.org/10.1210/er.2016-1146.

9. "Abdominal Fat and What to Do About It," Harvard Health Publishing. June 25, 2019, https://www.health.harvard.edu/staying-healthy/abdominal-fat-and-what-to-do-about-it.

10. J. Lambert, "Living Near Your Grandmother Has Evolutionary Benefits," NPR, https://www.npr.org/sections/goatsandsoda/2019/02/07/692088371/living-near-your-grandmother-has-evolutionary-benefits.

Chapter 2

1. Rahavi Gnanasegar, Wendy Wolfman, Leticia Hernandez Galan, Amie Cullimore, and Alison K. Shea, "Does Menopause Hormone Therapy Improve Symptoms of Depression? Findings from a Specialized Menopause Clinic," *Menopause* 31, no. 4 (2023): 320–25, https://doi.org/10.1097/gme.0000000000002325.

2. Jacques E. Rossouw, Ross L. Prentice, JoAnn E. Manson, LieLing Wu, David Barad, Vanessa M. Barnabei, Marcia Ko, Andrea Z. LaCroix, Karen L. Margolis, and Marcia L. Stefanick, "Postmenopausal Hormone Therapy and Risk of

Cardiovascular Disease by Age and Years Since Menopause," *JAMA* 297, no. 13 (2007): 1465–77, https://doi.org/10.1001/jama.297.13.1465.

3. Marianne Canonico, Emmanuel Oger, Geneviève Plu-Bureau, Jacqueline Conard, Guy Meyer, Hervé Lévesque, Nathalie Trillot, et al., "Hormone Therapy and Venous Thromboembolism Among Postmenopausal Women: Impact of the Route of Estrogen Administration and Progestogens: The ESTHER Study," *Circulation* 115, no. 7 (2007): 840–45, https://doi.org/10.1161/circulationaha.106.642280.

4. Haim A. Abenhaim, Samy Suissa, Laurent Azoulay, Andrea R. Spence, Nicholas Czuzoj-Shulman, and Togas Tulandi, "Menopausal Hormone Therapy Formulation and Breast Cancer Risk," *Obstetrics & Gynecology* 139, no. 6 (2022): 1103–10, https://doi.org/10.1097/aog.0000000000004723.

5. R. T. Chlebowski, G. L. Anderson, A. K. Aragaki, J. E. Manson, M. L. Stefanick, K. Pan, W. Barrington, L. H. Kuller, M. S. Simon, D. Lane, K. C. Johnson, T. E. Rohan, M. L. S. Gass, J. A. Cauley, E. D. Paskett, M. Sattari, & R. L. Prentice, "Association of Menopausal Hormone Therapy with Breast Cancer Incidence and Mortality During Long-Term Follow-up of the Women's Health Initiative Randomized Clinical Trials," *JAMA* 324, no. 4 (2020): 369–80. https://doi.org/10.1001/jama.2020.9482.

6. P. A. Van den Brandt, R. A. Goldbohm, and Valerie Berol, "Alcohol, Tobacco and Breast Cancer—Collaborative Reanalysis of Individual Data from 53 Epidemiological Studies, Including 58,515 Women with Breast Cancer and 95,067 Women Without the Disease," Collaborative Group on Hormonal Factors in Breast Cancer, *British Journal of Cancer* 87, no. 11 (2002): 1234–45, https://doi.org/10.1038/sj.bjc.6600596.

7. "NAMS Position Statement: The 2022 Hormone Therapy Position Statement of the North American Menopause Society," *Menopause* 29, no. 7 (2022): 767–94, https://www.menopause.org/docs/default-source/professional/nams-2022-hormone-therapy-position-statement.pdf.

8. Roger A. Lobo, James H. Pickar, John C. Stevenson, Wendy J. Mack, and Howard N. Hodis, "Back to the Future: Hormone Replacement Therapy as Part of a Prevention Strategy for Women at the Onset of Menopause," *Atherosclerosis* 254 (2016): 282–90, https://doi.org/10.1016/j.atherosclerosis.2016.10.005.

9. Ananthan Ambikairajah, Mizanur Khondoker, Edward Morris, Ann-Marie G. de Lange, Rasha NM Saleh, Anne Marie Minihane, and Michael Hornberger, "Investigating the Synergistic Effects of Hormone Replacement Therapy, Apolipoprotein E and Age on Brain Health in the UK Biobank," *Human Brain Mapping* 45, no. 2 (2024): e26612, https://doi.org/10.1002/hbm.26612.

10. Carolyn J. Crandall, Allison Diamant, and Nanette Santoro, "Safety of Vaginal Estrogens: A Systematic Review," *Menopause* 27, no. 3 (2020): 339–60, https://doi.org/10.1097/gme.0000000000001468; Pranjal Agrawal, Sajya M. Singh, Corey

Able, Kathryn Dumas, Jaden Kohn, Taylor P. Kohn, and Marisa Clifton, "Safety of Vaginal Estrogen Therapy for Genitourinary Syndrome of Menopause in Women with a History of Breast Cancer," *Obstetrics & Gynecology* 142, no. 3 (2023): 660–68, https://doi.org/10.1097/aog.0000000000005294; Lauren McVicker, Alexander M. Labeit, Carol A. C. Coupland, Blánaid Hicks, Carmel Hughes, Úna McMenamin, Stuart A. McIntosh, Peter Murchie, and Chris R. Cardwell, "Vaginal Estrogen Therapy Use and Survival in Females with Breast Cancer," *JAMA Oncology* 10, no. 1 (2024): 103–8, https://doi.org/10.1001/jamaoncol.2023.4508.

Chapter 3

1. G. A. Greendale, M. H. Huang, R. G. Wight, T. Seeman, C. Luetters, N. E. Avis, J. Johnston, and A. S. Karlamangla, "Effects of the Menopause Transition and Hormone Use on Cognitive Performance in Midlife Women," *Neurology* 72, no. 21 (2009): 1850–57.

2. G. A. Greendale, M. H. Huang, R. G. Wight, T. Seeman, C. Luetters, N. E. Avis, J. Johnston, and A. S. Karlamangla, "Effects of the Menopause Transition and Hormone Use on Cognitive Performance in Midlife Women," *Neurology* 72, no. 21 (2009): 1850–57, https://doi.org/10.1212/wnl.0b013e3181a71193.

3. Lorraine Dennerstein, John Randolph, John Taffe, Emma Dudley, and Henry Burger, "Hormones, Mood, Sexuality, and the Menopausal Transition," *Fertility and Sterility* 77 (2002): 42–48, https://doi.org/10.1016/s0015-0282(02)03001-7.

4. Nazanin E. Silver, "Mood Changes During Perimenopause Are Real. Here's What to Know," ACOG, April 2023, https://www.acog.org/womens-health/experts-and-stories/the-latest/mood-changes-during-perimenopause-are-real-heres-what-to-know.

5. Masakazu Terauchi, Tamami Odai, Asuka Hirose, Kiyoko Kato, Mihoko Akiyoshi, Mikako Masuda, Reiko Tsunoda, Hiroaki Fushiki, and Naoyuki Miyasaka, "Dizziness in Peri-and Postmenopausal Women Is Associated with Anxiety: A Cross-Sectional Study," *BioPsychoSocial Medicine* 12 (2018): 1–7, https://doi.org/10.1186/s13030-018-0140-1.

6. Jelena M. Pavlović, "Evaluation and Management of Migraine in Midlife Women," *Menopause* 25, no. 8 (2018): 927–29, https://doi.org/10.1097/GME.0000000000001104.

7. "Perimenopause: Rocky Road to Menopause," Harvard Health News, August 9, 2022, https://www.health.harvard.edu/womens-health/perimenopause-rocky-road-to-menopause.

8. Gabriela Kołodyńska, Maciej Zalewski, and Krystyna Rożek-Piechura, "Urinary Incontinence in Postmenopausal Women—Causes, Symptoms, Treatment," *Menopause Review* 18, no. 1 (2019): 46–50, https://doi.org/10.5114/pm.2019.84157.

9. Shen Lin, Hongjin Wang, Jingjing Qiu, Minghong Li, Ebin Gao, Xiaofeng Wu, Yunxiang Xu, and Guizhen Chen, "Altered Gut Microbiota Profile in Patients

with Perimenopausal Panic Disorder," *Frontiers in Psychiatry* 14 (2023): 1139992, https://doi.org/10.3389/fpsyt.2023.1139992.

10. "Perimenopause: Rocky Road to Menopause," Harvard Health News, August 9, 2022, https://www.health.harvard.edu/womens-health/perimenopause-rocky -road-to-menopause.

Chapter 4

1. Marianne Wessling-Resnick, "Iron Homeostasis and the Inflammatory Response," *Annual Review of Nutrition* 30, no. 1 (2010): 105–22, strokehttps://doi.org/10.1146 /annurev.nutr.012809.104804.

2. T. Mansour and Y. S. Chowdhury, *Endometrial Polyp*, updated April 25, 2023, in StatPearls (Internet) (StatPearls Publishing, January 2024), https://www.ncbi.nlm .nih.gov/books/NBK557824/.

3. Mie Jareid, Jean-Christophe Thalabard, Morten Aarflot, Hege M. Bøvelstad, Eiliv Lund, and Tonje Braaten, "Levonorgestrel-Releasing Intrauterine System Use Is Associated with a Decreased Risk of Ovarian and Endometrial Cancer, without Increased Risk of Breast Cancer. Results from the NOWAC Study," *Gynecologic Oncology* 149, no. 1 (2018): 127–32, https://doi.org/10.1016/j.ygyno.2018.02 .006.

4. Carolyn B. Sufrin, Debbie Postlethwaite, Mary Anne Armstrong, Maqdooda Merchant, Jacqueline Moro Wendt, and Jody E. Steinauer, "Neisseria Gonorrhea and Chlamydia Trachomatis Screening at Intrauterine Device Insertion and Pelvic Inflammatory Disease," *Obstetrics & Gynecology* 120, no. 6 (2012): 1314–21, http://10.1097/AOG.0b013e318273364c.

5. Mayisah Rahman, Connor King, Rosie Saikaly, Maria Sosa, Kristel Sibaja, Brandon Tran, Simon Tran, et al., "Differing Approaches to Pain Management for Intrauterine Device Insertion and Maintenance: A Scoping Review," *Cureus* 16, no. 3 (2024), https://doi.org/10.7759/cureus.55785.

6. S. Zeman, P. Havlík, J. Zemanová, and D. Němec, "Status of Bone Mineral Density After the Long-Standing Application of Contraception Depo-Provera," *Ceska Gynekologie* 78, no. 1 (2013): 116–24.

7. "Minipill (Progestin-Only Birth Control Pill)," Mayo Clinic, January 13, 2023, https://www.mayoclinic.org/tests-procedures/minipill/about/pac-20388306.

8. Florence Trémollieres, "Impact of Oral Contraceptive on Bone Metabolism," *Best Practice & Research Clinical Endocrinology & Metabolism* 27, no. 1 (2013): 47–53, https://doi.org/10.1016/j.beem.2012.09.002.

9. D. B. Cooper and P. Patel, *Oral Contraceptive Pills*, updated February 29, 2024, in StatPearls (Internet) (StatPearls Publishing, January 2024), available from https:// www.ncbi.nlm.nih.gov/books/NBK430882/.

10. L. A. Heinemann and J. C. Dinger, "Range of Published Estimates of Venous Thromboembolism Incidence in Young Women," *Contraception* 75, no. 5 (2007): 328–336. https://doi.org/10.1016/j.contraception.2006.12.018.

11. Y. Gorina, N. Elgaddal, and J. D. Weeks, "Hysterectomy Among Women Age 18 and Older: United States, 2021," NCHS Data Brief, no 494 (Hyattsville, MD: National Center for Health Statistics, 2024), https://dx.doi.org/10.15620/cdc:145592.

12. Farzaneh Kashefi, Marjan Khajehei, Mohammad Alavinia, Ebrahim Golmakani, and Javad Asili, "Effect of Ginger (*Zingiber officinale*) on Heavy Menstrual Bleeding: A Placebo-Controlled, Randomized Clinical Trial," *Phytotherapy Research* 29, no. 1 (2015): 114–19, https://doi.org/10.1002/ptr.5235.

Chapter 5

1. Haibin Li and Frank Qian, "Low-Risk Sleep Patterns, Mortality, and Life Expectancy at Age 30 Years: A Prospective Study of 172 321 US Adults," *Journal of the American College of Cardiology* 81, no. 8, Supplement (2023): 1675.

2. "AASM Sleep Prioritization Survey," American Academy of Sleep Medicine, 2023, https://aasm.org/wp-content/uploads/2023/06/sleep-prioritization-survey-2023 -waking-up-well-rested.pdf.

3. Yue Leng, Nick W. J. Wainwright, Francesco P. Cappuccio, Paul G. Surtees, Robert Luben, Nick Wareham, Carol Brayne, and Kay-Tee Khaw, "Self-Reported Sleep Patterns in a British Population Cohort," *Sleep Medicine* 15, no. 3 (2014): 295–302, https://doi.org/10.1016/j.sleep.2013.10.015.

4. James M. Trauer, Mary Y. Qian, Joseph S. Doyle, Shantha M. W. Rajaratnam, and David Cunnington, "Cognitive Behavioral Therapy for Chronic Insomnia: A Systematic Review and Meta-Analysis," *Annals of Internal Medicine* 163, no. 3 (2015): 191–204. https://doi.org/10.7326/M14-2841.

5. Ainissa Ramirez, *The Alchemy of Us* (MIT Press, 2020), 3–4.

6. Xiang Wang, Peihuan Li, Chen Pan, Lisha Dai, Yan Wu, and Yunlong Deng, "The Effect of Mind-Body Therapies on Insomnia: A Systematic Review and Meta-Analysis," *Evidence-Based Complementary and Alternative Medicine* 2019, no. 1 (2019): 9359807, https://doi.org/10.1155/2019/9359807.

7. Q. He, X. Chen, T. Wu, L. Li, and X. Fei, "Risk of Dementia in Long-Term Benzodiazepine Users: Evidence from a Meta-Analysis of Observational Studies," *Journal of Clinical Neurology* (Seoul, Korea) 15, no. 1 (2019): 9–19, https://doi.org/10.3988/jcn.2019.15.1.9.

Chapter 6

1. "Elektra Health's Annual Menopause in the Workplace Report (2022)—Elektra Health," Elektra Health, May 15, 2023, https://www.elektrahealth.com/workplace menopausesurvey/.

2. C. Hart-Kress, A. O'Sullivan, R. Hertel, and H. Hirsch, "Exploring Women's Top Fears About Menopausal Hormone Therapy in 2024," *Menopause* (December 2024).

3. "Early Onset Alzheimer's Disease," Johns Hopkins Medicine, retrieved October 8 from https://www.hopkinsmedicine.org/health/conditions-and-diseases /alzheimers-disease/earlyonset-alzheimer-disease.

4. "Women and Alzheimer's," Alzheimer's Association, https://www.alz.org/alzheimers -dementia/what-is-alzheimers/women-and-alzheimer-s, accessed February 28, 2025.

5. Gill Livingston, Jonathan Huntley, Kathy Y. Liu, Sergi G. Costafreda, Geir Selbæk, Suvarna Alladi, David Ames, et al., "Dementia Prevention, Intervention, and Care: 2024 Report of the Lancet Standing Commission," *Lancet* 404, no. 10452 (2024): 572–628.

6. Matilde Nerattini, Steven Jett, Caroline Andy, Caroline Carlton, Camila Zarate, Camila Boneu, Michael Battista, et al., "Systematic Review and Meta-Analysis of the Effects of Menopause Hormone Therapy on Risk of Alzheimer's Disease and Dementia," *Frontiers in Aging Neuroscience* 15 (2023): 1260427, https://doi.org /10.3389/fnagi.2023.1260427.

7. Robert Waldinger and Marc Schulz, *The Good Life: Lessons from the World's Longest Scientific Study of Happiness* (Simon and Schuster, 2023).

8. "Our Epidemic of Loneliness and Isolation: The U.S. Surgeon General's Advisory on the Healing Effects of Social Connection and Community," 2023, https:// www.hhs.gov/sites/default/files/surgeon-general-social-connection-advisory.pdf.

9. Hanne K. Collins, Serena F. Hagerty, Jordi Quoidbach, Michael I. Norton, and Alison Wood Brooks, "Relational Diversity in Social Portfolios Predicts Well-Being," *Proceedings of the National Academy of Sciences* 119, no. 43 (2022): e2120668119, https://doi.org/10.1073/pnas.2120668119.

10. Mark S. Granovetter, "The Strength of Weak Ties," *American Journal of Sociology* 78, no. 6 (1973): 1360–80.

11. L. Arab, R. Guo, and D. Elashoff, "Lower Depression Scores Among Walnut Consumers in NHANES," *Nutrients* 11, no. 2 (2019): 275, https://doi.org/10.3390 /nu11020275; F. Li, X. Liu, and D. Zhang, "Fish Consumption and Risk of Depression: A Meta-Analysis," *Journal of Epidemiology and Community Health* 70, no. 3 (2016): 299–304.

12. A. Evrensel and M. E. Ceylan, "The Gut-Brain Axis: The Missing Link in Depression," *Clinical Pharmacology and Neuroscience* 13, no. 3 (2015): 239–44, https://doi .org/10.9758/cpn.2015.13.3.239.

Chapter 7

1. M. Canonico, G. Plu-Bureau, G. D. Lowe, and P. Y. Scarabin, "Hormone Replacement Therapy and Risk of Venous Thromboembolism in Postmenopausal Women:

Systematic Review and Meta-analysis," *British Medical Journal (Clinical Research Ed.)* 336, no. 7655 (2008): 1227–31. https://doi.org/10.1136/bmj.39555.441944.BE.

2. S. Gopal, A. Ajgaonkar, P. Kanchi, A. Kaundinya, V. Thakare, S. Chauhan, and D. Langade, "Effect of an Ashwagandha (Withania Somnifera) Root Extract on Climacteric Symptoms in Women During Perimenopause: A Randomized, Double-Blind, Placebo-Controlled Study," *Journal of Obstetrics and Gynaecology Research* 47, no. 12 (2021): 4414–25, https://doi.org/10.1111/jog.15030.

3. M. Mehrpooya, S. Rabiee, A. Larki-Harchegani, A. M. Fallahian, A. Moradi, S. Ataei, and M. T. Javad, "A Comparative Study on the Effect of 'Black Cohosh' and 'Evening Primrose Oil' on Menopausal Hot Flashes," *Journal of Education and Health Promotion* 7, no. 36 (2018), https://doi.org/10.4103/jehp.jehp_81_17.

4. Neal D. Barnard, Hana Kahleova, Danielle N. Holtz, Tatiana Znayenko-Miller, Macy Sutton, Richard Holubkov, Xueheng Zhao, Stephanie Galandi, and Kenneth D. R. Setchell, "A Dietary Intervention for Vasomotor Symptoms of Menopause: A Randomized, Controlled Trial," *Menopause* 30, no. 1 (2023): 80–87, https://doi.org/10.1097/GME.0000000000002080.

5. Susan R. Davis and Sarah Wahlin-Jacobsen, "Testosterone in Women—the Clinical Significance," *Lancet Diabetes & Endocrinology* 3, no. 12 (2015): 980–92, https://doi.org/10.1016/s2213-8587(15)00284-3.

6. Shilpa N. Bhupathiraju, Francine Grodstein, Meir J. Stampfer, Walter C. Willett, Carolyn J. Crandall, Jan L. Shifren, and JoAnn E. Manson, "Vaginal Estrogen Use and Chronic Disease Risk in the Nurses' Health Study," *Menopause* 26, no. 6 (2019): 603–10, https://doi.org/10.1097/GME.0000000000001284.

7. Susan R. Davis, Rodney Baber, Nicholas Panay, Johannes Bitzer, Sonia Cerdas Perez, Rakibul M. Islam, Andrew M. Kaunitz, et al., "Global Consensus Position Statement on the Use of Testosterone Therapy for Women," *Journal of Sexual Medicine* 16, no. 9 (2019): 1331–37, https://doi.org/10.1210/jc.2019-01603.

8. Debra Herbenick, Michael Reece, Devon Hensel, Stephanie Sanders, Kristen Jozkowski, and J. Dennis Fortenberry, "Association of Lubricant Use with Women's Sexual Pleasure, Sexual Satisfaction, and Genital Symptoms: A Prospective Daily Diary Study," *Journal of Sexual Medicine* 8, no. 1 (2011): 202–12, https://doi.org/10.1111/j.1743-6109.2010.02067.x.

9. Jordan E. Rullo, Tierney Lorenz, Matthew J. Ziegelmann, Laura Meihofer, Debra Herbenick, and Stephanie S. Faubion, "Genital Vibration for Sexual Function and Enhancement: A Review of Evidence," *Sexual and Relationship Therapy* 33, no. 3 (2018): 263–74, https://doi.org/10.1080/14681994.2017.1419557.

Chapter 8

1. Giulia Menichetti, Babak Ravandi, Dariush Mozaffarian, and Albert-László Barabási, "Machine Learning Prediction of the Degree of Food Processing," *Nature Communications* 14, no. 1 (2023): 2312, https://doi.org/10.1038/s41467-023-37457-1.

2. Carlos Augusto Monteiro, Renata Bertazzi Levy, Rafael Moreira Claro, Inês Rugani Ribeiro de Castro, and Geoffrey Cannon, "Increasing Consumption of Ultra-Processed Foods and Likely Impact on Human Health: Evidence from Brazil," *Public Health Nutrition* 14, no. 1 (2011): 5–13, https://doi.org/10.1017/S1368980010003241.

3. Scheine Leite Canhada, Vivian Cristine Luft, Luana Giatti, Bruce Bartholow Duncan, Dora Chor, M. Maria de Jesus, Sheila Maria Alvim Matos, et al., "Ultra-Processed Foods, Incident Overweight and Obesity, and Longitudinal Changes in Weight and Waist Circumference: The Brazilian Longitudinal Study of Adult Health (ELSA-Brasil)," *Public Health Nutrition* 23, no. 6 (2020): 1076–86, https://doi.org/10.1017/S1368980019002854.

4. University of Connecticut Paul Rudd Center for Food Policy and Health, "Food Marketing," accessed January 24, 2024, from https://uconnruddcenter.org/research/food-marketing/.

5. K. L. Margolis, D. E. Bonds, R. J. Rodabough, L. Tinker, L. S. Phillips, C. Allen, T. Bassford, et al., "Effect of Oestrogen Plus Progestin on the Incidence of Diabetes in Postmenopausal Women: Results from the Women's Health Initiative Hormone Trial," *Diabetologia* 47 (2004): 1175–87, https://doi.org/10.1007/s00125-004-1448-x; S. R. Salpeter, J. M. E. Walsh, T. M. Ormiston, E. Greyber, N. S. Buckley, and E. E. Salpeter, "Meta-Analysis: Effect of Hormone-Replacement Therapy on Components of the Metabolic Syndrome in Postmenopausal Women," *Diabetes, Obesity and Metabolism* 8, no. 5 (2006): 538–54, https://doi.org/10.1111/j.1463-1326.2005.00545.x.

6. Katherin M. Flegal, Brian K. Kit, Heather Orpana, and Barry I. Graubard, "Association of All-Cause Mortality with Overweight and Obesity Using Standard Body Mass Index Categories: A Systematic Review and Meta-Analysis," *JAMA* 309, no. 1 (2013): 71–82, https://doi.org/10.1001/jama.2012.113905.

7. Shoaib Afzal, Anne Tybjærg-Hansen, Gorm B. Jensen, and Børge G. Nordestgaard, "Change in Body Mass Index Associated with Lowest Mortality in Denmark, 1976–2013," *JAMA* 315, no. 18 (2016): 1989–96, https://doi.org/10.1001/jama.2016.4666.

8. Nathan R. Weeldreyer, Jeison C. De Guzman, Craig Paterson, Jason D. Allen, Glenn A. Gaesser, and Siddhartha S. Angadi, "Cardiorespiratory Fitness, Body Mass Index and Mortality: A Systematic Review and Meta-Analysis," *British Journal of Sports Medicine* (2024), https://doi.org/10.1136/bjsports-2024-108748.

9. D. Arterburn, T. Sofer, D. M. Boudreau, A. Bogart, E. O. Westbrook, M. K. Theis, G. Simon, and S. Haneuse, "Long-Term Weight Change After Initiating Second-Generation Antidepressants," *Journal of Clinical Medicine* 5, no. 4 (2016): 48, https://doi.org/10.3390/jcm5040048.

10. Lisa Buss Preszler, "Health Benefts of Semaglutide—Beyond Weight Loss," Mayo Clinic Press, July 2, 2024, https://mcpress.mayoclinic.org/living-well/health-benefits-of-semaglutide-beyond-weight-loss/.

11. Irza Wajid, Alexis Vega, Katherine Thornhill, Jack Jenkins, Chandler Merriman, Debbie Chandler, Sahar Shekoohi, Elyse M. Cornett, and Alan D. Kaye, "Topiramate (Topamax): Evolving Role in Weight Reduction Management: A Narrative Review," *Life* 13, no. 9 (2023): 1845, https://doi.org/10.3390/life13091845.

12. Erin Fothergill, Juen Guo, Lilian Howard, Jennifer C. Kerns, Nicolas D. Knuth, Robert Brychta, Kong Y. Chen, et al., "Persistent Metabolic Adaptation 6 Years After 'The Biggest Loser' Competition," *Obesity* 24, no. 8 (2016): 1612–19, https://doi.org/10.1002/oby.21538.

13. Jean-Pierre Montani, A. K. Viecelli, Anne Prévot, and Abdul G. Dulloo, "Weight Cycling During Growth and Beyond as a Risk Factor for Later Cardiovascular Diseases: The 'Repeated Overshoot' Theory," *International Journal of Obesity* 30, no. 4 (2006): S58–S66.

14. Huajie Zou, Ping Yin, Liegang Liu, Wu Duan, Pu Li, Yan Yang, Wenjun Li, Qunchuan Zong, and Xuefeng Yu, "Association Between Weight Cycling and Risk of Developing Diabetes in Adults: A Systematic Review and Meta-Analysis," *Journal of Diabetes Investigation* 12, no. 4 (2021): 625–32.

15. Matthew A. Cottam, Heather L. Caslin, Nathan C. Winn, and Alyssa H. Hasty, "Multiomics Reveals Persistence of Obesity-Associated Immune Cell Phenotypes in Adipose Tissue During Weight Loss and Weight Regain in Mice," *Nature Communications* 13, no. 1 (2022): 2950.

16. Ghada A. Soliman, "Dietary Fiber, Atherosclerosis, and Cardiovascular Disease," *Nutrients* 11, no. 5 (2019): 1155, https://doil.org/10.3390/nu11051155; Marc P. McRae, "Dietary Fiber Intake and Type 2 Diabetes Mellitus: An Umbrella Review of Meta-Analyses," *Journal of Chiropractic Medicine* 17, no. 1 (2018): 44–53, https://doi.org/10.1016/j.jcm.2017.11.002.

17. Elena Jovanovski, Shahen Yashpal, Allison Komishon, Andreea Zurbau, Sonia Blanco Mejia, Hoang Vi Thanh Ho, Dandan Li, John Sievenpiper, Lea Duvnjak, and Vladimir Vuksan, "Effect of Psyllium (Plantago Ovata) Fiber on LDL Cholesterol and Alternative Lipid Targets, Non-HDL Cholesterol and Apolipoprotein B: A Systematic Review and Meta-Analysis of Randomized Controlled Trials," *American Journal of Clinical Nutrition* 108, no. 5 (2018): 922–32, https://doi.org/10.1093/ajcn/nqy115.

18. Zeinab Gholami, Cain C. T. Clark, and Zamzam Paknahad, "The Effect of Psyllium on Fasting Blood Sugar, HbA1c, HOMA IR, and Insulin Control: A GRADE-Assessed Systematic Review and Meta-Analysis of Randomized Controlled Trials," *BMC Endocrine Disorders* 24 (2024), https://doi.org/10.1186/s12902-024-01608-2.

19. Y. Mavros, N. Gates, G. C. Wilson, N. Jain, J. Meiklejohn, H. Brodaty, W. Wen, N. Singh, B. T. Baune, C. Suo, M. K. Baker, N. Foroughi, Y. Wang, P. S. Sachdev, M. Valenzuela, and M. A. Fiatarone Singh, "Mediation of Cognitive Function Improvements by Strength Gains After Resistance Training in Older Adults with Mild Cognitive Impairment: Outcomes of the Study of Mental and Resistance Training," *Journal of the American Geriatrics Society* 65, no. 3 (2017): 550–59, https://doi.org/10.1111/jgs.14542; P. J. O'Connor, M. P. Herring, and A. Caravalho, "Mental Health Benefits of Strength Training in Adults," *American Journal of Lifestyle Medicine* 4, no. 5 (2010): 377–96.

20. Glenn N. Levine, Karen Allen, Lynne T. Braun, Hayley E. Christian, Erika Friedmann, Kathryn A. Taubert, Sue Ann Thomas, Deborah L. Wells, and Richard A. Lange, "Pet Ownership and Cardiovascular Risk: A Scientific Statement from the American Heart Association," *Circulation* 127, no. 23 (2013): 2353–63.

21. "Having a Dog Can Help Your Heart—Literally," Harvard Health Publishing, September 1, 2015, https://www.health.harvard.edu/staying-healthy/having-a-dog-can-help-your-heart--literally.

Chapter 9

1. National Center for Health Statistics, "Multiple Cause of Death 2018–2021 on CDC WONDER Database," accessed February 2, 2023. https://wonder.cdc.gov/mcd.html.

2. Katherine Harmon Courage, "How Menopause Affects Cholesterol—and How to Manage It," *Time*, September 21, 2022, https://time.com/6215450/how-menopause-affects-cholesterol/.

3. Roger A. Lobo, James H. Pickar, John C. Stevenson, Wendy J. Mack, and Howard N. Hodis, "Back to the Future: Hormone Replacement Therapy as Part of a Prevention Strategy for Women at the Onset of Menopause," *Atherosclerosis* 254 (2016): 282–90, https://doi.org/10.1016/j.atherosclerosis.2016.10.005.

4. Samar R. El Khoudary, Brooke Aggarwal, Theresa M. Beckie, Howard N. Hodis, Amber E. Johnson, Robert D. Langer, Marian C. Limacher, et al., "Menopause Transition and Cardiovascular Disease Risk: Implications for Timing of Early Prevention: A Scientific Statement from the American Heart Association," *Circulation* 142, no. 25 (2020): e506–e532, https://doi.org/10.1161/CIR.0000000000000912.

5. Grishma Hirode and Robert J. Wong, "Trends in the Prevalence of Metabolic Syndrome in the United States, 2011–2016," *JAMA* 323, no. 24 (2020): 2526–28, https://doi.org/10.1001/jama.2020.450.1.

6. Sarah A. Burgard and Jennifer A. Ailshire, "Gender and Time for Sleep Among US Adults," *American Sociological Review* 78, no. 1 (2013): 51–69, https://doi.org/10.1177/0003122412472048.

7. Consensus Conference Panel, Nathaniel F. Watson, M. Safwan Badr, Gregory Belenky, Donald L. Bliwise, Orfeu M. Buxton, Daniel Buysse, et al., "Recommended Amount of Sleep for a Healthy Adult: A Joint Consensus Statement of the American Academy of Sleep Medicine and Sleep Research Society," *Journal of Clinical Sleep Medicine* 11, no. 6 (2015): 591–92, https://doi.org/10.5664/jcsm.4758.

8. Shahrad Taheri, Ling Lin, Diane Austin, Terry Young, and Emmanuel Mignot, "Short Sleep Duration Is Associated with Reduced Leptin, Elevated Ghrelin, and Increased Body Mass Index," *PLoS medicine* 1, no. 3 (2004): e62, https://doi.org/10.1371/journal.pmed.0010062.

9. Rebecca C. Thurston, Yuefang Chang, Christopher E. Kline, Leslie M. Swanson, Samar R. El Khoudary, Elizabeth A. Jackson, and Carol A. Derby, "Trajectories of Sleep Over Midlife and Incident Cardiovascular Disease Events in the Study of Women's Health Across the Nation," *Circulation* 149, no. 7 (2024): 545–55, https://doi.org/10.1161/CIRCULATIONAHA.123.066491.

10. Rebecca Robbins, Stuart F. Quan, Matthew D. Weaver, Gregory Bormes, Laura K. Barger, and Charles A. Czeisler, "Examining Sleep Deficiency and Disturbance and Their Risk for Incident Dementia and All-Cause Mortality in Older Adults Across 5 Years in the United States," *Aging* 13, no. 3 (2021): 3254, https://doi.org/10.18632/aging.202591.

11. Borja del Pozo Cruz, Matthew Ahmadi, Sharon L. Naismith, and Emmanuel Stamatakis, "Association of Daily Step Count and Intensity with Incident Dementia in 78 430 Adults Living in the UK," *JAMA Neurology* 79, no. 10 (2022): 1059–63, https://doi.org/10.1001/jamaneurol.2022.2672.

12. Elizabeth Mostofsky, I-Min Lee, Julie Elizabeth Buring, and Kenneth Jay Mukamal, "Impact of Alcohol Consumption on Breast Cancer Incidence and Mortality: The Women's Health Study," *Journal of Women's Health* (2024), https://doi.org/10.1089/jwh.2023.1021.

13. Noelle K. LoConte, Abenaa M. Brewster, Judith S. Kaur, Janette K. Merrill, and Anthony J. Alberg, "Alcohol and Cancer: A Statement of the American Society of Clinical Oncology," *Journal of Clinical Oncology* 36, no. 1 (2018): 83–93.

14. Office of the Surgeon General, "Alcohol and Cancer Risk: The U.S. Surgeon General's Advisory," 2025, https://www.hhs.gov/sites/default/files/oash-alcohol-cancer-risk.pdf.

Chapter 10

1. Maha S. A. Abdel Hadi, "Sports Brassiere: Is It a Solution for Mastalgia?," *Breast Journal* 6, no. 6 (2000): 407–9.

2. Roseane B. de Miranda, Patrícia Weimer, and Rochele C. Rossi, "Effects of Hydrolyzed Collagen Supplementation on Skin Aging: A Systematic Review and Meta-Analysis," *International Journal of Dermatology* 60, no. 12 (2021): 1449–61.

3. Shiloah A. Kviatkovsky, Robert C. Hickner, Hannah E. Cabre, Stephanie D. Small, and Michael J. Ormsbee, "Collagen Peptides Supplementation Improves Function, Pain, and Physical and Mental Outcomes in Active Adults," *Journal of the International Society of Sports Nutrition* 20, no. 1 (2023): 2243252, https://doi.org/10.1080/15502783.2023.2243252

4. Seok Hyun Bae, Young Joo Shin, Ha Kyoung Kim, Joon Young Hyon, Won Ryang Wee, and Shin Goo Park, "Vitamin D Supplementation for Patients with Dry Eye Syndrome Refractory to Conventional Treatment," *Scientific Reports* 6, no. 1 (2016): 33083.

5. Zeying Chen, Chengxiao Zhang, Jiaxuan Jiang, Junwen Ouyang, Di Zhang, Taige Chen, Yiran Chu, and Kai Hu, "The Efficacy of Vitamin D Supplementation in Dry Eye Disease: A Systematic Review and Meta-Analysis," *Contact Lens and Anterior Eye* (2024): 102169, https://doi.org/10.1016/j.clae.2024.102169.

6. Jisha K. Pillai and Venkataram Mysore, "Role of Low-Level Light Therapy (LLLT) in Androgenetic Alopecia," *Journal of Cutaneous and Aesthetic Surgery* 14, no. 4 (2021): 385–91, https://doi.org/10.4103/JCAS.JCAS_218_20.

7. Kevin R. Brough and Rochelle R. Torgerson, "Hormonal Therapy in Female Pattern Hair Loss," *International Journal of Women's Dermatology* 3, no. 1 (2017): 53–57, https://doi.org/10.1016/j.ijwd.2017.01.001.

8. Y. Nestoriuc and A. Martin, *Efficacy of Biofeedback for Migraine: A Meta-Analysis*, 2007, in Database of Abstracts of Reviews of Effects (DARE): Quality-Assessed Reviews, internet, York (UK): Centre for Reviews and Dissemination (UK); 1995, available from https://www.ncbi.nlm.nih.gov/books/NBK73546/.

9. Ji-yong Bae, Hyun-Kyung Sung, Na-Yoen Kwon, Ho-Yeon Go, Tae-jeong Kim, Seon-Mi Shin, and Sangkwan Lee, "Cognitive Behavioral Therapy for Migraine Headache: A Systematic Review and Meta-Analysis," *Medicina* 58, no. 1 (2021): 44, https://doi.org/10.3390/medicina58010044.

10. Fatemeh Sharifzadeh, Maryam Kashanian, Jalil Koohpayehzadeh, Fatemeh Rezaian, Narges Sheikhansari, and Nooshin Eshraghi, "A Comparison Between the Effects of Ginger, Pyridoxine (Vitamin B6) and Placebo for the Treatment of the First Trimester Nausea and Vomiting of Pregnancy (NVP)," *Journal of Maternal-Fetal & Neonatal Medicine* 31, no. 19 (2018): 2509–14.

11. Masakazu Terauchi, Tamami Odai, Asuka Hirose, Kiyoko Kato, Mihoko Akiyoshi, Mikako Masuda, Reiko Tsunoda, Hiroaki Fushiki, and Naoyuki Miyasaka,

"Dizziness in Peri- and Postmenopausal Women Is Associated with Anxiety: A Cross-Sectional Study," *BioPsychoSocial Medicine* 12 (2018): 1–7.

12. Dana Henry, "Causes of Dizziness During Menopause," *Medical News Today*, updated May 8, 2024, https://www.medicalnewstoday.com/articles/319860.

Chapter 11

1. R. A. Lobo, J. H. Pickar, J. C. Stevenson, W. J. Mack, and H. N. Hodis, "Back to the Future: Hormone Replacement Therapy as Part of a Prevention Strategy for Women at the Onset of Menopause," *Atherosclerosis* 254 (2016): 282–90, https://doi.org/10.1016/j.atherosclerosis.2016.10.005.

2. Alex Janin, "Your Healthspan Is as Important as Your Lifespan—and It's Declining," *Wall Street Journal*, updated January 17, 2024, https://www.wsj.com/health/wellness/americans-unhealthy-chronic-disease-3f35c9f5.

3. Andrew Bazeley, Catherine Marren, and Alex Shepherd, "Menopause and the Workplace," Fawcett Society, 2022, https://www.fawcettsociety.org.uk/menopause andtheworkplace.

4. Gill Livingston, Jonathan Huntley, Kathy Y. Liu, Sergi G. Costafreda, Geir Selbæk, Suvarna Alladi, David Ames, et al., "Dementia Prevention, Intervention, and Care: 2024 Report of the Lancet Standing Commission," *Lancet* 404, no. 10452 (2024): 572–628.

5. Jun-Mo Kim, Tae-Hee Kim, Hae-Hyeog Lee, Seung Hun Lee, and Tong Wang, "Postmenopausal Hypertension and Sodium Sensitivity," *Journal of Menopausal Medicine* 20, no. 1 (2014): 1–6, https://doi.org/10.6118/jmm.2014.20.1.1.

6. Heather Currie and Christine Williams, "Menopause, Cholesterol and Cardiovascular Disease," *US Cardiology* 5, no. 1 (2008): 12–14.

7. Yejin Kim, Yoosoo Chang, In Young Cho, Ria Kwon, Ga-Young Lim, Jae Hwan Jee, Seungho Ryu, and Mira Kang, "The Prevalence of Thyroid Dysfunction in Korean Women Undergoing Routine Health Screening: A Cross-Sectional Study," *Thyroid* 32, no. 7 (2022): 819–27, https://doi.org/10.1089/thy.2021.0544.

8. Endocrine Society, "Menopause and Bone Loss," January 23, 2022, https://www.endocrine.org/patient-engagement/endocrine-library/menopause-and-bone-loss.

9. David G. Blanchflower and Andrew J. Oswald, "Is Well-Being U-Shaped Over the Life Cycle?," *Social Science & Medicine* 66, no. 8 (2008): 1733–49, https://doi.org/10.1016/j.socscimed.2008.01.030; Christoph Wunder, Andrea Wiencierz, Johannes Schwarze, and Helmut Küchenhoff, "Well-Being Over the Life Span: Semiparametric Evidence from British and German Longitudinal Data," *Review of Economics and Statistics* 95, no. 1 (2013): 154–67, https://www.jstor.org/stable/23355657.

10. Katherine E. Campbell, Lorraine Dennerstein, Mark Tracey, and Cassandra E. Szoeke, "The Trajectory of Negative Mood and Depressive Symptoms over Two Decades," *Maturitas* 95 (2017): 36–41.

11. Social Issues Research Centre, "Jubilee Women. Fiftysomething Women—Lifestyle and Attitudes Now and Fifty Years Ago," http://www.sirc.org/publik/jubilee-women.pdf.

12. Jack Zenger and Joseph Folkman, "How Age and Gender Affect Self-Improvement," *Harvard Business Review*, 2016, https://hbr.org/2016/01/how-age-and-gender-affect-self-improvement.

13. Lisa Mosconi, *The Menopause Brain* (Avery, 2024), 98–99.

Appendix A

1. F. Mauvias-Jarvis, J. Manson, J. Stevenson, and V. Fonseca, "Menopausal Hormone Therapy and Type 2 Diabetes Prevention: Evidence, Mechanisms, and Clinical Implications," *Endocrine Reviews* 28, no. 3 (2017): 173–88.

2. Mark Messina, "Impact of Soy Foods on the Development of Breast Cancer and the Prognosis of Breast Cancer Patients," *Research in Complementary Medicine* 23, no. 2 (2016): 75–80, https://doi.org/10.1159/000444735.

3. Roger A. Lobo, James H. Pickar, John C. Stevenson, Wendy J. Mack, and Howard N. Hodis, "Back to the Future: Hormone Replacement Therapy as Part of a Prevention Strategy for Women at the Onset of Menopause," *Atherosclerosis* 254 (2016): 282–90.

4. Shilpa N. Bhupathiraju, Francine Grodstein, Meir J. Stampfer, Walter C. Willett, Carolyn J. Crandall, Jan L. Shifren, and JoAnn E. Manson, "Vaginal Estrogen Use and Chronic Disease Risk in the Nurses' Health Study," *Menopause* 26, no. 6 (2019): 603–10, https://doi.org/10.1097/gme.0000000000001284.

5. Pranjal Agrawal, Sajya M. Singh, Corey Able, Kathryn Dumas, Jaden Kohn, Taylor P. Kohn, and Marisa Clifton, "Safety of Vaginal Estrogen Therapy for Genitourinary Syndrome of Menopause in Women with a History of Breast Cancer," *Obstetrics & Gynecology* 142, no. 3 (2022): 660–68, https://doi.org/10.1097/aog.0000000000005294.

INDEX

abdominal fat, 18, 157

abnormal uterine bleeding, 69–70. *See also* heavy bleeding

acne, 53, 86, 211, 216–17

acupuncture, 230, 231, 263

Addyi (flibanserin), 125–26, 152, 264

adenomyosis, 58, 71, 75

ADHD medications and libido, 148

Adipex, 171–73

age, myth of being too young for perimenopause, 24–25

alcohol, 30, 182, 204–7
  cancer risk and, 41, 205
  health risks of, 119, 144, 204–7, 236
  hot flashes and, 143, 144
  medications for addiction, 171
  sleep and, 98, 111–12, 206

allergies, 53, 225, 232

Alzheimer's disease. *See* early-onset Alzheimer's

anemia, 71, 72, 79

annual physicals, 251–54

anovulation, 77

anticonvulsants, 165

antidepressants, 7–8, 28–29, 105–6, 143, 148, 165

antifungals, 148, 241

antihistamines, 148, 165, 226

antipsychotics, 165

antiseizure medications, 149

anxiety, 4, 53, 58, 207–8
  causes of, 94, 96–98

health-care-related, 98–100

medications, 28, 29, 105–6, 114, 148

nighttime. *See* "lying awake and worrying" symptom set

perimenopausal symptoms vs., 29, 36, 53, 56

supplements for, 130

weight gain and, 168, 169, 172

appetite-suppressant medications, 171–73

arthritis, 17, 122, 193

artificial tears, 224

ashwagandha, 139, 144, 223

autoimmune diseases, 43, 117, 122–23

Aygestin, 102

back pain, 4, 56, 91, 184–85

balance
  clumsiness, 223–24
  exercises, 201, 223–24

balayam, 229

bariatric surgery, 86, 256

beans and legumes, 142, 176, 177, 178–79, 203, 217

bedroom environment, 107, 108–9, 182, 224

bedtime routine, 107–8

"bedtime yoga," 110

belladonna, 91

benzodiazepine, 113–14

beta-blockers, 149, 165

beverages, 50, 182–83, 202

"Biggest Loser" model, 173–74

bioidentical hormone therapy, 44, 46, 83, 100–102, 268
birth control, 9, 84–87, 267–68. *See also* combined oral contraceptives; Depo-Provera; progesterone-only oral birth control
contraindications, 86–87
heavy bleeding and, 75, 82–85
hormone therapy vs., 42, 267–68
libido and, 149
myths and misconceptions, 31, 42
side effects, 85–86
weight gain and, 165, 265
black cohosh, 91, 139, 144
"bleeding 'til you drop" symptom set. *See* heavy bleeding
bloating, 53, 102, 217–18
fiber and diet, 178, 217–18
blood circulation, 154–55, 198
blood clots, 43, 86, 89, 138, 204
blood pressure. *See* high blood pressure
blood sugar, 19, 20, 33, 95, 131, 160, 191–92, 231, 253
blood tests, 27, 78, 123, 135, 252–54
blood thinners and heavy bleeding, 76
blue light, 108, 130
body image, 160, 163–64
body odor, 53, 133, 135, 142, 232
body temperature, 13–14, 55, 97, 102, 108, 138, 221, 264
bone density, 16, 17, 187, 193
DXA scans, 210, 256–57
bone fractures, xv, 17, 45, 187
bone health, 85, 193–94, 197, 198, 257
brain, xv, 259
estrogen and, 11, 15, 121
neuroplasticity, 117, 152–53, 182
progesterone and, 12
brain fog, 4, *10*, 53, 58, 116–21, 135–45. *See also* "dragging yourself through life" symptom set; "feeling unrecognizable" symptom set

at-home remedies for, *140*, 140–42
cognitive decline vs., 193
treatments for, 135–39
brain health, 192–93
diet for, 131, 212
exercise for, 198, 199
hormone therapy for, 45–46
bra size, 157
breast cancer, ix, xv, 7, 99, 193
family history of, 42, 43, 46, 269
hormone therapy and, 39–43, 46, 87, 205
mammogram screenings, 7, 254–55
progesterone-only birth control, 86
breastfeeding, 21, 119
breast tenderness, 53, 86, 99, 124, 218–19
breathing exercises, 112–13, 144, 233
Brisdelle (paroxetine salt), 139, 143, 263–64
brittle nails, 53, 72, 219–20
burning feet, 221–22

caffeine, 94, 111, 143, 236
calcium, 212, 219, 228, 257
caloric consumption, 174–75
"calories in, calories out" model, 174, 182–83
cancer. *See also* breast cancer; uterine cancer
alcohol and, 41, 205
hormone-sensitive, 270
obesity and, 163
screenings, 254–56
carbohydrates, 158, 160, 203
cardio exercise, 180–81, 200–201
cardio health. *See* heart health
cardiovascular (heart) disease, xv, 190–91
estrogen and, 16, 18, 190
hormone therapy and, 38, 39, 40, 45, 87, 150, 191
loneliness and, 128–29
metabolic syndrome and, 19–20, 192
semaglutides and, 170
sleep and, 95
weight and diet, 158, 163, 174

cardiovascular system and estrogen and, xv, 16, 17
care team, 248, 248–50
celiac disease, 122
cervix, 46–47, 73–74, 88
  IUD insertion, 79, 80, 81–82
chamomile, 231
chin hairs, 222–23
cholesterol, 43, 59, 187, 190–91
  estrogen and, 18, 20
  exercise and, 198
  screening, 166, 252–53
  sleep and, 95
  weight and diet, 162, 164, 170, 178, 180, 185, 203, 204
chronic fatigue syndrome, 22, 116, 117, 122, 126, 136, 245
circadian rhythms, 107–8, 130
clitoris, 19, 46–47, 145, 151, 194
clumsiness, 223–24
cognitive behavioral therapy (CBT), 100, 125, 127, 141–42, 144, 230, 260
cognitive behavioral therapy for insomnia (CBT-I), 104–5, 109–10, 275
cognitive decline, 28, 95, 116–17, 192–93. See also dementia; early-onset Alzheimer's
cold hands or feet, 72, 219
collagen, 54, 57, 176, 219, 220
  supplements, 220–21
colonoscopies, 255–56
combined oral contraceptives, 31, 85, 87, 126–27, 143, 268
  contraindications, 87
  side effects, 86
complete blood count (CBC), 78, 136
conjugated equine estrogen (CEE), 38–41
constipation, 11, 71, 74, 168, 172, 180, 217, 226, 236, 237, 254
cortisol, 33–34, 59, 108, 222
couples counseling, 154
COVID-19, 128–29, 232. See also long COVID

cramps, 71, 75, 79, 80, 90, 92, 211
cranberry juice, 238
C-reactive protein (CRP), 136

dementia, xv, 118–19, 192–93, 244, 278. See also early-onset Alzheimer's
  exercise for, 198, 200
  loneliness and, 128–29
  sleep and, 113–14, 196
dentists, 249
Depo-Provera, 82–83, 86, 165
depression, 29, 36, 120–21, 207–8
  alcohol and, 206
  diet for, 131
  herbal remedies for, 91, 130
  hormone therapy for, 29
  medications, 7–8, 28–29, 105–6, 143, 148, 165, 244
  perimenopausal symptoms vs., 29, 36
  postpartum, 44, 119
  serotonin and, 27
  sleep and, 95
  weight gain and, 161
dermatologists, 216–17
diabetes, 192
  diet for, 160
  estrogen and, 17–20, 234
  hormone therapy and, 40, 43, 45, 87, 137, 160–61
  medications, 7, 165, 168
  uterine cancer and, 76
  weight gain and, 160–61, 163
diet, 50–51, 174–80, 202–7
  appetite-suppressant medications, 171–73
  caloric consumption, 174–75
  for dizziness, 235
  fats in, 202–3
  fermented foods in, 131, 237, 241
  for hair, 228–29
  for heart health, 190–91
  heavy bleeding, 91

diet *(cont.)*
for nausea, 231
omega-3 fatty acids in, 131, 204, 212
portion sizes, 159–60, 174–75
protein in, 130–31, 175–80, 202–3,
228–29
for rage, 233
self-assessment, 209
for skin health, 226
ultra-processed foods in, 158–59, 202
for vasomotor symptoms, 142
weight and, 156, 158, 159–60, 162, 164,
173–80
digestion. *See also* bloating
diet and probiotics for, 112, 178, 203, 204
exercise for, 217
hydration for, 183
digestive system and estrogen, 17–18, 102
dilation and curettage (D&C), 73–74, 75
diuretics, 149, 229, 234, 236
dizziness, 14, 54–55, 72, 234–35
doctor consultation, 64–66, 268
fill-in-the-blank script for, 281–82
doctors, menopause-certified, 6, 249, 272,
273–74
dogs, health benefits of, 183
dopamine, 125–26, 130, 197, 260, 264
dopamine agonists, 125–26, 139, 152,
167–68
"dragging yourself through life" symptom
set, 58, 115–31
at-home remedies for, *127*, 127–31
autoimmune conditions, 122–23
brain fog and depression, 120–21
causative factors of, 118
misdiagnosis, 117
motherhood and, 119–20
symptoms of, 118
treatments for, 123–27
drowsiness, 98, 102, 103, 107, 109–10, 114,
226
dry and itchy skin, 15, 56, 58, 72, 225–27, 254

dry eyes, 15, 35, 224–25
dry mouth, 53–54, 196
Dutch Test, 26–27

early-onset Alzheimer's, xiv, 22, 99, 117,
118–19, 193, 278
ears. *See also* tinnitus
dry and itchy, 225, 226
estrogen and, 14, 234
ectopic pregnancies, 80–81
endometrial ablation, 87
endometrial cancer, 80, 87
endometriosis, 58, 71, 72, 75
endorphins, 128, 197, 232–33
estradiol, 102–4, 142
hormone therapy, 40, 41, 43, 44, 79–80,
83, 85, 101, 102–4, 123–24, 136, 142, 268
for weight gain, 166–67
estrogen, 4, *10*, 11–12, 21–22
brain fog and depression, 116–17, 120–21
from head to toe, 14–19
heavy bleeding and, 70
hormonal hallmarks, *10*
insulin resistance and, 160–61
libido and, 145–46
metabolic syndrome and, 18, 19–21
myths and misconceptions about,
25–28, 30, 33–34, 36–42, 44–48
screening, 26, 27, 78
sleeplessness and, 97, 98
thirty-four symptoms, 52–58
estrogen therapy. *See specific therapies*
evening primrose oil, 218
exercise, 127–28, 140–41, 180–82, 197–201
for balance, 201, 223–24
for blood circulation, 154–55
for digestion, 217
for heart health, 180, 198
for incontinence, 237
for mood, 127–28, 198
overexercising, 173–74
for rage, 232–33

self-assessment, 209
for stress, 127–28, 197–98, 200, 201, 232–33
types of, 199–201
for weight, 161, 162, 164, 167, 173–74, 180–82
exogenous hormones, 42
eyes
dry. See dry eyes
estrogen and, 15

fatigue, 22, 25, 55, 58, 94, 231. See also chronic fatigue syndrome; "dragging yourself through life" symptom set
anemia and, 72
estrogen and, 14
weight gain and, 161, 162
fat phobia, 160, 162, 163–64
fats, 203–4
fecal occult blood tests, 255–56
"feeling unrecognizable" symptom set, 58–59, 132–55
at-home remedies for, 140, 140–42
causative factors of, 134
libido, 145–55
symptoms of, 134
treatments for, 133–34, 135–39
Female Sexual Function Index (FSFI), 147–48
Femring, 83, 138
fermented foods, 131, 237, 241
fertility, xxi, 31, 74, 266
fezolinetant, 138–39, 143, 264
fiber, 50, 131, 142, 158, 160, 175–80, 203, 217–18
high-fiber foods, list, 178–79
fibroids, 18, 58, 69, 74–75, 88
fibromyalgia, 116, 117, 126, 245
financial health, 246–47
flexibility, exercises, 201
follicle-stimulating hormone (FSH), 6, 10, 13

blood tests, 26, 27, 78, 123, 271
levels, 13, 271
follicular phase, 35
food. See diet
frequently asked questions (FAQs), 263–72
friendships, 128–29, 207

gamma-aminobutyric acid (GABA), 94, 97, 113, 232
gas, 217–18
genitourinary health, 194–95
genitourinary syndrome of menopause (GSM), 19, 42, 149, 194–95, 240, 263
genitourinary (GU) tract, 19, 46–47, 48, 150
ghrelin, 162, 169, 196
ginger, 90, 231
glucagon-like peptide-1 (GLP-1), 169–71
glucose, 20, 21, 37, 57, 123, 160, 161, 164, 169, 177, 180, 185, 186–87, 191–92, 197
gonadotropinreleasing hormone (GnRH), 75
grandmother hypothesis, 21
gratitude, 207, 233, 260
gut bacteria (gut microbiome), 57, 131, 168, 177, 180, 208, 217
gynecologists, 249

hair and estrogen, 14
hair care, 227, 228
hair changes, 54, 227–28
hair loss, 79, 216, 228–29
hair masks, 227
"hangry," 131, 178, 233
happiness, 258–60
Hashimoto's disease, 122
Haver, Mary Claire, 129, 277
headaches (migraines), 55, 99, 230
anemia and, 72
diet for, 202
estrogen and, 121, 202
exercise for, 201
hormone therapy and, 49, 87, 137, 230

headaches (migraines) *(cont.)*
  medications, 165, 230
  remedies for, 130, 230
  sleep apnea and, 196
health-care-related anxiety, 98–100
heart attacks, 43, 97, 170, 183, 191, 196, 270
heart disease. *See* cardiovascular disease
heart failure medications, 149
heart health, 190–91
  exercise for, 180, 198
  sleep and, 196
heart palpitations, 3–4, 16, 29, 54, 56, 58, 97,
    103, 231, 235
heavy bleeding, 21, 55, 58, 63, 69–92
  anatomical factors contributing to,
    73–76
  at-home remedies for, 89, 90–92
  causative factors of, 71
  hormonal factors of, 70
  medications causing, 76
  other possible contributing factors, 77
  progesterone and, 55, 70
  symptoms of, 70–71
  treatments for, 77–89, 142, 143
herbal remedies, 90, 139, 144, 218, 231
high blood pressure (hypertension),
    190–91
  exercise for, 198
  hormone therapy and, 43, 87, 137, 167, 191
  medications, 149, 170, 236
  screening, 20, 251–52
  sleep and, 95
  uterine cancer and, 76
  weight and, 163
histamine, 53, 225
hormones, xvi–xvii, 3–23. *See also specific
    hormones*
  cast of characters, 11–14
  "reproductive," 4–8
  sleep and, 97
  symptoms, 10, 21–22
  thirty-four symptoms, 52–58

hormone-sensitive cancer, 270
hormone therapy (HT). *See also specific
    therapies*
  begin date of, 272
  birth control vs., 42, 267–68
  breast cancer and, 39–43, 46, 205
  contraindications, 43–44
  doctor consultation, 65–66
  dosage, 269
  for "dragging yourself through life"
    symptom set, 123–25
  effects, how long, 265
  end date, 269
  FAQs, 263–72
  fertility and, 31
  for "feeling unrecognizable" symptom
    set, 136–38
  for heart health, 191
  for heavy bleeding, 78–82, 83
  for hot flashes, 42, 135–38, 142–43
  for libido, 149–51
  for "lying awake and worrying"
    symptom set, 100–104
  myths and misconceptions about,
    38–42, 44–48
  for silent symptoms, 210–11
  systemic vs. local, 83, 84
  for weight gain, 166–68, 265
hot flashes, 35, 55, 135–45
  at-home remedies for, 143–44
  burning feet and, 221
  estrogen volatility and, 97, 98
  hormone therapy for, 42, 135–38, 142–43
  medications for, 143, 263–64
  self-hypnosis for, 110–11, 144, 275
  treatments for, 135–39, 142–44
human papillomavirus (HPV) tests, 255
humidifiers, 224, 232
hyaluronic acid, 238
hydration, 91–92, 111, 144, 182–83, 217, 218,
    219, 226, 231, 235–38, 240
hypothalamus, 11, 15, 33, 55, 143, 264

hypothyroidism, 14, 122–23
hysterectomies, 31, 75, 88–89, 267

incontinence, 55, 118, 125, 187, 194, 235–37
inner ears, 14, 54, 223, 234–35
insomnia. *See* "lying awake and worrying"
   symptom set; sleep disturbances
insulin, 18, 160–61, 160, 186–87,
   191–92, 197
iron levels, 91
iron-rich foods, 220
irritability, xvii, 12, 36, 56, 58, 94. *See also*
   "feeling unrecognizable" symptom set
itchy skin. *See* dry and itchy skin
IUDs (intrauterine devices), xvii, 83. *See*
   also progesterone-releasing IUDs
   heavy bleeding and, 76, 77, 89
   myths and misconceptions, 31, 80–81
   nonhormonal, 76, 80
   painful insertion, 80, 81–82

joint aches and pain, 4, 16–17, 56, 58, 193,
   244–45
joints, exercise for, 127–28, 197,
   199–200, 201

kegels, 154, 236
keratin, 53, 54, 219
kidney dysfunction, 17, 136, 171
klonopin, 113–14
kombucha, 112, 217, 241

labia, 19, 46–47, 237
leptin, 162, 172, 196
L-glutamine, 226
libido, 6, 54, 125–26, 145–55
   at-home remedies for, 152–55, *153*
   medications for, 264
   medications for low, 152
   medications lowering, 148–49
   testosterone and, 12–13
   treatments, 135–36, 148, 149–52

life expectancy, 21, 45, 95, 163
life satisfaction, 258–60
lifespan and hormonal fluctuations,
   35–36, *36*
lightheadedness, 72, 235
liver, 18, 41, 98, 169
liver disease, 43, 86, 87, 136, 170, 187
loneliness, 128–29, 183
long COVID, 4–5, 116, 132, 136
lubes, 153–54, 239
lungs and estrogen, 16
luteal phase, 35, 83, 124
luteinizing hormone (LH), 82–83, 126
"lying awake and worrying" symptom set,
   58, 93–114
   at-home remedies for, *106,* 106–13
   causative factors of, 94, 96–98
   medications for, 113–14
   risks of, 95–98
   symptoms of, 57, 94
   treatments for, 100–106
Lyme disease, 116

magnesium glycinate, 110, 223
makeup, 216
mammograms, 7, 254–55
masturbation, 154
medical school training, xviii–xix, 4
medications, 7–8. *See also specific*
   medications
Mediterranean-style diet, 202, 205
medroxyprogesterone acetate (MPA),
   39, 82
melatonin, 98, 108
menopause
   definition of, 9
   diagnostic criterion, xvi
   hormone levels, xvi–xvii
   myths and misconceptions, 30–31
   symptoms and hormonal hallmarks, *10*
   use of term, ix–xi
menopause retreats, 129

menopause transition, 9
  symptoms and hormonal hallmarks, *10*
menstrual cramps, 71, 75, 79, 80, 90, 92, 211
mental health, 207–8. *See also* anxiety;
    depression; mood
  myths and misconceptions about,
    27–28, 36–37
  self-assessment, 209
metabolic health, 51, 167, 191–92
metabolic syndrome, 18, 19–21, 95, 191–92
metabolism, 37–38, 174–75
  estrogen and, 18
  thyroid hormones and, 13–14
metformin, 168, 253
migraines. *See* headaches
minoxidil, 229
miscarriages, 77, 78
misdiagnosis, 117, 244
moisturizers (moisturizing), 219, 225,
    226, 232
  vaginal, 238, 239
mood (mood changes), 56, 86, 207–8, 244.
    See also irritability; rage
  antidepressants and perimenopausal
    symptoms, 28–29
  exercise for, 127–28, 198
  hormone therapy, 136
  myths about hormones and, 27–28,
    36–37
  progesterone and, 12
  weight gain and, 161
Mosconi, Lisa, 121, 259, 277
motherhood, 119–20
multiple endocrine neoplasia syndrome
    type 2 (MEN 2), 171
muscle aches, 56, 134, 201
muscle mass, 185, 187, 193–94, 202
  protein for, 202
  strength training for, 200, 202
  testosterone and, 12–13, 150
  weight gain and, 161–62
myths and misconceptions, xx, 24–49

nail polish, 219, 220
nails, brittle. *See* brittle nails
nausea, 86, 231
navigating the transition, 243–61
nervous system, 112–13
  breathing for, 144
  cortisol and, 33
  estrogen and, 15–16, 55
neuroplasticity, 117, 152–53, 182
night sweats, 35, 56, 64, 132
  burning feet and, 221
  estrogen volatility and, 97, 98
  hormone therapy for, 42, 102–3, 136,
    245, 247
  treatments for, 104, 136, 138–39, 144, 275
nighttime anxiety and insomnia. *See*
    "lying awake and worrying"
    symptom set
nitric oxide, 16, 17
norethindrone, 84–85, 143, 268
novelty-seeking, 141, 147, 152–53
NSAIDs (nonsteroidal anti-inflammatory
    drugs), 17, 72, 234
nutritionists, 183–84, 250
NuvaRing, 83, 126

obesity, 76, 162–63. *See also* weight gain
omega-3 fatty acids, 131, 204, 212
organ prolapse, 19, 187, 194
Osphena, 264
osteoclasts, 16, 257
osteoporosis, 193
ovaries, removal, 266–67
Ozempic, 164, 169–71

painful sex, 47, 145, 239–40
  fibroids and, 75
  pelvic floor and, 154, 236
  symptoms and, 54, 57, 64, 194
  vaginal estrogen and, 47, 125, 136,
    149, 240
panic attacks, 56–57, 97, 113

panty liners, 241
Pap smears, 255
"peezing," 235–36
pelvic floor, 19, 47, 55, 237
    exercises, 154, 236
pelvic inflammatory disease (PID), 81
perimenopause
    author's story, xvii–xviii
    definition of, 8
    diagnostic criterion, xvi, 5–6
    hormones and, 3–23
    long tentacles of, xv
    myths and misconceptions, xx, 24–49
    remedies not recommended, 32–33
    symptoms and hormonal hallmarks, 10
    symptoms assessment, xx, 50–62
    symptom sets, xx, 51–52, 58–59, 67–212
    two phases of, 8–9, 10
period, 5–6
    heavy bleeding. See heavy bleeding
    hormonal fluctuations, 35–36
    irregular, 25, 29, 31, 56, 63, 86, 91, 122
    last menstrual (LMP), 6, 42, 210
    myths and misconceptions about, 25, 29,
        30–31, 44–46
    phases of perimenopause, 8–9, 10
    sleep and, 101, 103
    tracking cycles, 22–23, 35–36, 48–49, 61,
        65, 77–78, 211
peripheral neuropathy, 221
personal trainers, 250
pets, health benefits of, 183
phantom smells, 232
physical therapists, 250
pineal gland, 107–8
pituitary glands, 11, 13
placebo, 38–41, 85, 90, 126, 223
placebo effect, 33, 101, 265
pleasure, lack of, 54, 58, 118, 141
PMS, 25, 42
polycystic ovary syndrome (PCOS), 76, 77
polyps, 58, 73–74, 255–56

post-menopause
    definition, 9
    symptoms and hormonal hallmarks, 10
prebiotics, 217
pregnancy, 4
    myths and misconceptions about
        perimenopause and, 31
    progesterone and, 12
pregnancy tests, 3, 78
Premarin, 38–41
premenstrual dysphoric disorder (PMDD),
    42, 44–46
Prempro, 39–41
probiotics, 112, 217, 237, 266
progesterone, 4, 12, 35
    heavy bleeding and, 55, 70, 71, 76
    hormonal hallmarks, 10
    myths and misconceptions about, 27–28,
        30, 34, 39
    screening, 78
    sleep and, 97
    symptoms assessment, 53, 55, 56, 58–59
progesterone-only oral birth control
    ("mini pill"), 79, 84–85, 86, 102, 143,
        267–68
    contraindications, 86
    side effects, 86
progesterone-releasing IUDs, 9, 78–81, 83,
    124, 210–11
    myths and misconceptions about, 31,
        80–81
    painful insertion, 81–82
    for silent symptoms, 210–11
progesterone therapy, 39–41, 44–46, 124.
    See also combined oral contraceptives;
        progesterone-only oral birth control;
        progesterone-releasing IUDs
    hot flashes and, 142
    for "lying awake and worrying"
        symptom set, 100–102, 103
    side effects, 101–2
    for weight gain, 166–67

Prometrium, 41, 44, 83, 100–102, 268
protein, 130–31, 175–80, 202–3, 228–29
  high-protein foods, list, 177
psyllium, 180

Qsymia, 171–73
quercetin, 226

rage, 56, 232–33
Ramirez, Ainissa, 109
raspberry leaf tea, 90
red meat, 176, 177, 190, 202, 253
"reproductive" hormones, 4–8
retirement, 246–47
rhodiola, 130
romantasy, 141

saliva, 53–54
scalp, 227–28
schedule, consistency in, 107–8
screenings, 250–57
  misconception about, 25–27
seasonal affective disorder (SAD), 130
self-care, 30, 32, 194–95, 245–46
self-hypnosis, 110–11, 144, 263, 275
self-stimulation, 154
self-talk, 141–42, 160
semaglutide medications, 164,
    169–71, 253
serotonin, 263, 264
  estrogen and, 15, 27, 53, 56, 230, 232
  gut bacteria and, 131
  migraines and, 230
  rage and, 232
sex. See libido
sex hormone-binding globulin (SHBG), 14
sexual desire, 153. See also libido
sexual dysfunction, 54
sexually transmitted diseases (STDs), 77,
    78, 187, 194, 240
sexual satisfaction, 245
shampoos, 227–28

silent symptoms, 59, 186–212. See also
    specific symptoms
  at-home remedies for, 211, 211–12
  causative factors of, 188
  four pillars of health, 195–209
  hallmarks of, 187–88
  treatments for, 210–11
skin, 225–27
  dry and itchy. See dry and itchy skin
  elasticity, 15, 56, 57
  estrogen and, 15
skin care, 216, 225–26, 240
skin-care products, 216
sleep, 27, 51, 195–97
  benefits of, 95, 195–96
  building good habits, 96, 98, 107–10, 182
  for chin hairs, 222–23
  exercise for, 198
  medications, 7–8, 98, 113–14
  for migraines, 230
  myths and misconceptions about, 32,
    33–34
  self-assessment, 209
sleep apnea, 163, 196
  warning signs, 196
sleep disturbances (insomnia), 58, 95–98,
    195–96, 275. See also "lying awake and
    worrying" symptom set
  alcohol and, 98, 111–12, 206
  at-home remedies for, 106–13
  causes of, 94, 96–98
  hormone therapy, 44, 45
  as symptom of perimenopause, 57, 94
  weight gain and, 161, 166–67, 170
sleep hunger, 103, 109
sleep restriction, 109–10
smell sensitivity, 54, 232
smoking, 30, 43, 87, 205, 220, 221, 252
snoring, 16, 108–9, 196
SNRIs (serotoninnorepinephrine reuptake
    inhibitors), 105–6
sodas, 182–83, 202

solo symptoms, 215–42. *See also specific symptoms*
sore nipples, 218–19
soy, 130, 139, 142, 266
spicy foods, 143, 231
sports bras, 218
spotting, 49, 85, 86
SSRIs (selective serotonin reuptake inhibitors), 105–06, 139, 143
steroids, 117, 165
strength training, 128, 140, 180–82, 199–200
stress. *See also* "lying awake and worrying" symptom set
   exercise for, 127–28, 197–98, 200, 201, 232–33
   remedies for, 110–13, 130, 141–42, 144, 183, 207–8, 222–23, 230, 232–33
   sleep and hormones, 33–34, 51, 133
stress incontinence, 55, 236
stretching, 101, 110, 126, 140, 201
strokes, xv, 20, 40, 87, 170, 183, 192, 193, 196, 252, 270
suicidal thoughts, 29
sunlight, 130
sun protection, 130, 226
supplemental estrogen, 80, 102, 123–24, 230
supplements, 130, 139, 144. *See also specific supplements*
symptoms, xiv, xv, xxi, 8, *10. See also specific symptoms*
   FAQs, 270–71
   hormones and, 3–5, 21–22
symptoms assessment, xx, 50–62
   charting your course, 59–62
   doctor consultation, 64–66
   symptom sets, 58–59
   thirty-four symptoms, 52–58
   tracking, 22–23, 35–36, 48–49, 59–60, 77–78, 100, 141, 211, 243
symptom sets, xx, 51–52, 58–59, 67–212. *See also specific sets*
   75 percent rule, 63

synthetic progestin, 41, 42, 84, 85, 102, 143, 268
Synthroid, 14, 122–23
systemic hormone therapy, 83, *84,* 151, 270

tamoxifen, 76
targeted treatments, 142, 215–42
taste, changes in, 53–54
tea tree oil, 241
temporomandibular joint (TMJ), 234
testosterone, 12–13, 86, 222
   libido and, 145–46, 150–51
   screening, 26, 27
   weight gain and, 161–62
therapists, 3, 93, 96, 100, 250, 274–75
therapy. *See* cognitive behavioral therapy
thyroid function
   low, 77, 117
   screening, 253–54
thyroid hormones, 13–14, 78
   synthetic (Synthroid), 14, 122–23
thyroid-stimulating hormone (TSH), 78
tinnitus, 14, 57, 168, 233–34
tiredness. *See* "dragging yourself through life" symptom set; fatigue
topical vaginal estrogen, 149–50, 240
total iron-binding capacity (TIBC), 78
tracking symptoms, 22–23, 35–36, 48–49, 59–60, 77–78, 100, 141, 211, 243
transdermal estrogen, 41, 126, 137–38, 151, 247, 268, 270
triglycerides, 190–91
triptans, 230

ultra-processed foods, 158–59, 202
undereating, 173–74
Unlock Your Menopause Type (Hirsch), xvi, 188, 278
urethra, 18–19, 46, 57, 238
urinary incontinence. *See* incontinence
urinary tract and estrogen, 18–19

urinary tract infections (UTIs), 47, 57, 99, 187, 237–39
uterine artery embolization (UAE), 87–88
uterine cancer, xiv, 72, 75–76, 88, 101, 103, 124, 210–11
uterine fibroids, 18, 58, 74–75, 88
uterus, 39, 71, 75
  estrogen and, 18
  polyps, 73–74

vagina
  estrogen and, 19
  myths and misconceptions, 46–48
vaginal bleeding, unexplained, 43
vaginal dryness, 57, 86, 167, 194, 211, 239–40
vaginal estrogen, 47–48, 124–25, 149–50, 211, 238, 270
vaginal moisturizers, 238, 239
vaginal rings, 83–84, 124, 138
vegetables, 91, 142, 167, 178, 178–79, 190, 202, 203, 204, 226, 240, 252
Veozah (fezolinetant), 138–39, 143, 264
vertigo, 14, 223–24, 234–35
vestibulitis, 235
vitamin B6, 219, 231
vitamin B12, 130, 221–22, 228
vitamin C, 91, 226, 228, 240–41
vitamin D, 123, 130, 212, 224, 257
vitamin E, 238, 239
vulva, 19, 46–47, 145, 151, 194, 270
Vyleesi (bremelanotide), 152, 264

waist size, 20, 157, 158, 164, 185
water retention, 86, 218, 221
weak ties, 129
Wegovy, 164, 169–71
weight and estrogen, 15, 18
weight gain, 57–58, 59, 86, 156–85, 187–88
  at-home remedies for, 173, 173–84
  causative factors of, 158–59
  health risks of, 162–64
  hormone therapy and, 166–68, 265
  link between perimenopause and, 160–62
  medications causing, 165
  myths and misconceptions, 37–38
  symptoms, 157
  treatments, 166–73
weight loss
  at-home remedies for, 173, 173–84
  treatments, 166–73
weight training. See strength training
Wellbutrin (bupropion), 125–26, 139, 167–68
white noise, 107, 108–9, 234
Winfrey, Oprah, xiiii–xiv, 30
work and work-life balance, 34, 61, 246–47
wrinkles, 15, 220–21

yarrow, 90
yeast infections, 240–41
yoga, 110, 140, 155, 181, 197, 199, 201, 222–23, 224, 229

zinc, 232
"zingers," 15–16, 55

ABOUT THE AUTHOR

Heather Hirsch, MD, MS, MSCP, is the CEO and founder of The Collaborative by Heather Hirsch, MD, a private telemedicine practice focused on treating women at midlife, and the Heather Hirsch Academy, a platform dedicated to training health-care professionals about women's health. She is also co-building an AI-based menopause company, RealDocAI, with the mission to improve access to care.

Before starting her private practice, Dr. Hirsch founded the Menopause and Midlife Clinic at the Brigham and Women's Hospital and served on the faculty at Harvard Medical School. She is board-certified in internal medicine and completed the advanced fellowship training in women's health at the Cleveland Clinic. Dr. Hirsch is an active contributing member of the Menopause Society and the International Society for the Study of Women's Health, and has been featured on *Oprah Daily*, *The Drew Barrymore Show*, *Live with Kelly and Mark*, and in the *New York Times*.

Also the author of *Unlock Your Menopause Type*, and a prolific social media educator with a large, passionate following, Dr. Hirsch is on a mission to support the millions of women going through the menopause transition and to improve access to treatment for all women in midlife. Connect with her across social media @heatherhirschmd.

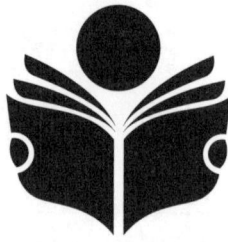

RAISING READERS
Books Build Bright Futures

Thank you for reading this book and for being a reader of books in general. As a author, I am so grateful to share being part of a community of readers with yo and I hope you will join me in passing our love of books on to the next generatic of readers.

Did you know that reading for enjoyment is the single biggest predictor of child's future happiness and success?

More than family circumstances, parents' educational background, or incom reading impacts a child's future academic performance, emotional well-bein communication skills, economic security, ambition, and happiness.

Studies show that kids reading for enjoyment in the US is in rapid decline:

- In 2012, 53% of 9-year-olds read almost every day. Just 10 years later, in 2022, the number had fallen to 39%.
- In 2012, 27% of 13-year-olds read for fun daily. By 2023, that number was just 14%.

Together, we can commit to **Raising Readers** and change this trend. How?

- Read to children in your life daily.
- Model reading as a fun activity.
- Reduce screen time.
- Start a family, school, or community book club.
- Visit bookstores and libraries regularly.
- Listen to audiobooks.
- Read the book before you see the movie.
- Encourage your child to read aloud to a pet or stuffed animal.
- Give books as gifts.
- Donate books to families and communities in need.

RQR1217

Books build bright futures, and **Raising Readers** is our shared responsibility.

For more information, visit **JoinRaisingReaders.com**

Sources: National Endowment for the Arts, National Assessment of Educational Progress, WorldBookDay.org, Nielsen BookData's 2023 "Understanding the Children's Book Consumer"